Surgical Treatment of Astigmatism

Surgical Treatment of Astigmatism

James P. Gills, MD
St. Luke's Cataract and Laser Institute
Tarpon Springs, Florida

Robert G. Martin, MD
Carolina Eye Associates
Southern Pines, North Carolina

Spencer P. Thornton, MD, FACS
Thornton Eye Surgery Center
Nashville, Tennessee

Donald R. Sanders, MD, PhD
Center for Clinical Research
Chicago, Illinois

Medical Writer
Project Coordinator
Michelle A. Van Der Karr

SLACK Incorporated, 6900 Grove Road, Thorofare, NJ 08086-9447

Publisher: John H. Bond
Managing Editor: Amy E. Drummond
Project Editor: Peter T. Christy

Surgical treatment of astigmatism/edited by James P. Gills . . .(et al.).
    p. cm.
    Includes bibliographical references and index.
    ISBN 1-55642-220-2
    1. Astigmatism—surgery.   I. Gills, James P.
    (DNLM: 1. Astigmatism—surgery   WW 310 S961 1994.
    RC932.S85   1994
    617.7'55--dc20
    DNLM/DLC   94-856
    for Library of Congress   CIP

Printed in the United States of America

Published by: SLACK Incorporated
               6900 Grove Road
               Thorofare, NJ 08086-9447

Last digit is print number: 10 9 8 7 6 5 4 3 2 1

To my patients, to my staff, and to my family:
That they may have better sight and insight for those
things both distant and near (multifocal corneas and souls)

"Where there is no vision, the people perish."
(Proverbs 29:18)

Jim Gills

Contents

Chapter 8
Corneal Transplantation and Astigmatic Keratotomy
Robert G. Martin, MD

Section III Wound Management Techniques in Cataract Surgery

Chapter 9
Cataract Incisions at the Steep Axis
Johnny L. Gayton, MD
Patrick Rowan, MD
Michelle A. Van Der Karr

Chapter 10
Keratolenticuloplasty
Robert M. Kershner, MD

Section IV Intraocular Lens Correction

Chapter 11
Clinical Investigation of a Toric IOL: FDA Study Update
Donald R. Sanders, MD, PhD
Manus C. Kraff, MD
John Shepherd, MD
Harry B. Grabow, MD

Index

Contributing Authors

Daniel S. Durrie, MD, Associate Clinical Professor, University of Missouri–Kansas City, Kansas City, Missouri

Johnny L. Gayton, MD, EyeSight Associates of Middle Georgia, Warner Robins, Georgia

James P. Gills, MD, Clinical Professor, University of South Florida, Tampa, Florida, St. Luke's Cataract and Laser Institute, Tarpon Springs, Florida

Harry B. Grabow, MD, Medical Director, Sarasota Cataract Institute, Director of Research and Education, International Cataract Foundation, Inc., Sarasota, Florida, Clinical Assistant Professor, University of South Florida, Tampa, Florida

R. Bruce Grene, MD, Grene Cornea, P.A., Assistant Clinical Professor, Department of Surgery, University of Kansas School of Medicine–Wichita, Wichita, Kansas

Don Johnson, MD, Medical Director, London Place Eye Centre, New Westminster, British Columbia

Robert M. Kershner, MD, FACS, Associate Clinical Professor, Department of Ophthalmology, University of Utah Medical Center, Salt Lake City, Utah, Chief, Section of Ophthalmology, Northwest Hospital, Director, Orange Grove Eye Surgery Center, Tucson, Arizona

Colman R. Kraff, MD, Clinical Instructor in Ophthalmology, Northwestern University, Chicago, Illinois

Manus C. Kraff, MD, Professor of Clinical Ophthalmology, Northwestern University, Chicago, Illinois

Richard L. Lindstrom, MD, Clinical Professor of Ophthalmology, University of Minnesota, Attending Surgeon, Phillips Eye Institute, Minneapolis, Minnesota

Robert G. Martin, MD, Director, Medical Care International Ophthalmic Research and Training Institute, Founder, Carolina Eye Associates, Southern Pines, North Carolina

Patrick Rowan, MD, Director, Rowan Eye Center, New Port Richey, Florida

Donald R. Sanders, MD, PhD, Associate Professor of Ophthalmology, University of Illinois at Chicago Eye Center, Director, Center for Clinical Research, Chicago, Illinois

D. James Schumer, MD, Fellow, Cornea and Refractive Surgery, Hunkeler Eye Clinic, Kansas City, Missouri

John Shepherd, MD, Associate Clinical Professor of Ophthalmology, University of Utah, Medical Director, Shepherd Eye Center, Las Vegas, Nevada

Alan V. Spigelman, MD, Sinai Hospital, William Beaumont Hospital, Detroit, Michigan

Roger F. Steinert, MD, Harvard Medical School, Center for Eye Research, Ophthalmic Consultants of Boston, Boston, Massachusetts

Vance M. Thompson, MD, Assistant Clinical Professor, University of South Dakota, School of Medicine, Sioux Falls, South Dakota

Spencer P. Thornton, MD, FACS, Director, Thornton Eye Surgery Center, Nashville, Tennessee

Michelle A. Van Der Karr, Center for Clinical Research, Chicago, Illinois

Preface

Recent advances in ophthalmology have led to heightened expectations among patients. Many patients wish to dispense with glasses and contacts and demand excellent uncorrected acuity. Given this environment, there has been a surging of interest in the correction of astigmatic errors, whether in the penetrating keratoplasty patient, the cataract patient, or the refractive patient. New techniques, improved nomograms, new diagnostic methods, and better surgical equipment have made astigmatism correction safer and more predictable. Computerized videokeratography, or corneal topography, permits a better understanding of the nature of the astigmatism preoperatively and the effect of surgery on the entire corneal shape. Laser technology, still in its infancy with regard to refractive correction, promises a new frontier. And, the toric intraocular lens promises to relieve astigmatism without affecting the corneal surface.

This book discusses some of the currently available methods of correcting astigmatism. None of these methods provide the answer for every patient, but all promise a partial or total alleviation of this visually disabling disorder.

Section I

Refractive Techniques

1

Background and Theory of Corneal Relaxing Incisions

SPENCER P. THORNTON, MD, FACS

Introduction

Following a number of false starts over the years, modern corneal refractive surgery was introduced to the United States in 1978 by Svyatoslov Fyodorov[1] and Leo Bores.[2] Since that time a number of studies have verified the relative safety and efficacy of incisional keratotomy for the correction of myopia and astigmatism. Today the progressive ophthalmologist has added astigmatic keratotomy (AK) with corneal relaxing incisions (CRIs) to his surgical armamentarium for all types of astigmatism.

Refractive surgery for congenital and surgically induced astigmatism is now recognized as a "natural" consequence of recent developments in technology and instrumentation, with new diamond micrometer knives, accurate to the hundredth of a millimeter, and corneal topography devices offering a means of planning and following corneal surgery with unprecedented accuracy. Most important has been a greater understanding of the physiology of the incised cornea and the predictability of effect of altered corneal curvature.

The Effect of Adding and Removing Tissue

The cornea may be made steeper by removing tissue, as in wedge resection, or by tight suture closure following cataract surgery. As the cornea becomes steeper, the radius of curvature is reduced and the refractive power increased in the steepened meridian, reflecting the increased power.

The cornea is made flatter by adding tissue, and an unsutured incision acts as if tissue is added by relaxation of the incised tissue. The radius of curvature is increased, and the keratometric reading and the refractive power are reduced in the flattened meridian.

To understand the basis for these effects, we shall look at the background and theoretical basis for corneal relaxing incisions.

The Barrier Principle - Theory and Application

An incision in the cornea always acts as if tissue is added. The tissue is "added" or "relaxed" at right angles to the direction of the incision (Figure 1-1). If the incision is placed radially, its action is transmitted 360° around the circumference of the cornea, provided there are no "barriers." In the usual radial keratotomy (RK), the first incision (and the second incision, if opposite the first) increases the circumference 360° (Figure 1-2). An incision placed 90° away from the first and second incisions (i.e., halfway between the first and second incisions) acts over an area of 180°, that is, 90° to either side of that incision, until it hits the previously placed incisions which act as a "barrier" (Figure 1-3A). Any subsequently added incisions have their action between adjacent incisions (Figure 1-3B).

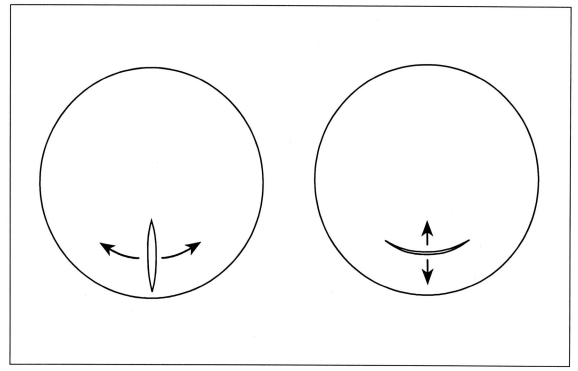

Figure 1-1. Relaxing incisions act as if tissue is added, and the radius of curvature is increased at right angles to the incision.

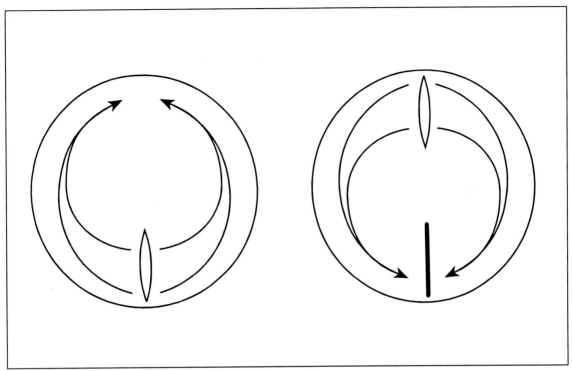

Figure 1-2. Corneal circumference is increased 360° with first two incisions.

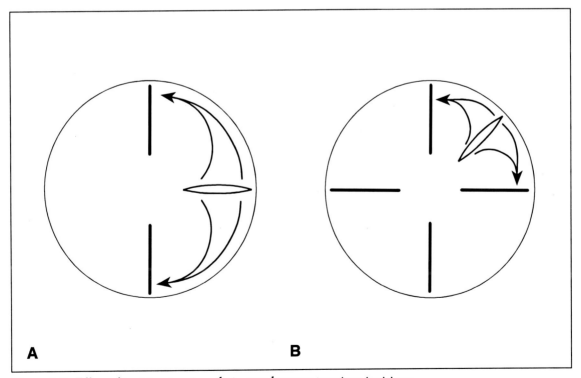

Figure 1-3. Effect of incision is primarily in area between previous incisions.

Transverse relaxing incisions, whether straight "T" incisions or arcuate incisions, "add tissue" in the meridian across which they are placed (remember, the action produced by an incision is at right angles to the incision). The reason that these incisions are so powerful is that their circumferential effect is limited and therefore concentrated by a "limiting barrier," the limbus (Figure 1-4).

Barrier Tissue

Congruous tissue transmits forces of relaxation or tension uniformly unless impaired in some way. If there is any interference by a "barrier" or discontinuity, this uniformity will be interrupted. Tissues non-congruous to the corneal stroma are the limbus and any scars that may be present in the cornea.

The interface of host and donor tissue after penetrating keratoplasty (PKP) becomes an "artificial limbus," interrupting the continuity and uniformity of the corneal tissue, and will limit the transmission of relaxation of tissue produced by corneal relaxing incisions placed in the donor button to within the donor button itself. Because the area of congruous tissue is smaller, an incision of any given length in a PKP button will have more effect than similar incisions placed in a "virgin" cornea.

Another incision crossing the path of the "effect area" also acts as a barrier. This barrier may impede the effect or enhance it depending on the direction of the incision. When that incision is

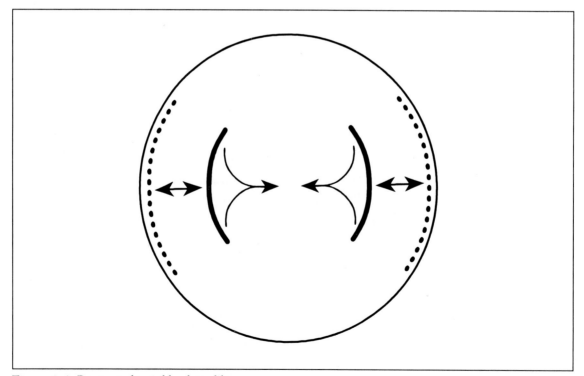

Figure 1-4. Barrier indicated by dotted line.

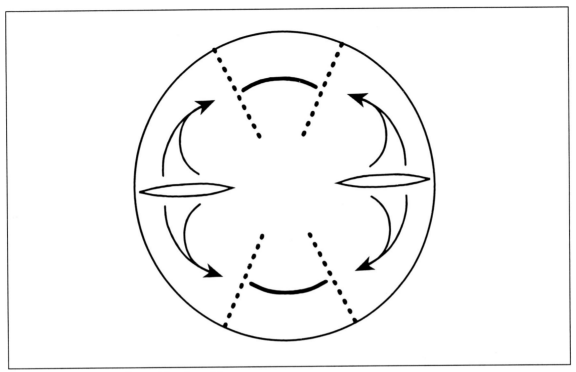

Figure 1-5. Barrier indicated by dotted lines.

in the same direction (as with additional radial incisions) the effect is enhanced between the incisions. When the incision is at right angles to the primary incision, the effect is impeded or restricted (as in the case of combined T incisions and radials) (Figure 1-5).

The Hinge Theory

Some authors have stated that the flattening effect across the meridian of steeper corneal curvature with "T" incisions occurs because of a "hinge" effect of arcuate incisions placed equidistant from the corneal apex. This hinge supposedly pushes tissue from the concave side of the arcuate incision toward the apex of the corneal dome and occurs because the base of the chord of the arcuate incision acts as a "hinge" (Figure 1-6). I believe this concept is in error.

More accurately, since tissue is effectively added with any incision, no matter what its curvature or lack of it, the "added tissue" is at right angles to the incision, and in the meridian of steep curvature across the corneal dome, the effect of increased circumference is limited by the limbus to a "band" across the cornea, the meridional corneal diameter. The limbus thus acts as a "barrier" and confines the effect of the relaxing incisions primarily to the area between the incisions (see Figure 1-4), much as a megaphone magnifies sound confined within the walls of the megaphone.

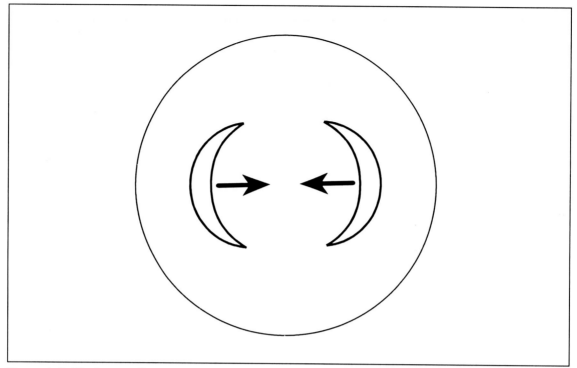

Figure 1-6. The hinge effect.

This confining of the effect of arcuate incisions acts to magnify the effect, and accounts for the fact that these incisions are so powerful for any given length. We have found clinically that up to 2.5 D astigmatism can be corrected with only one arcuate incision across the steep meridian (on the steeper side as indicated by corneal topography), aiming at slight undercorrection (Gills, personal communication).

Coupling

Whereas radial incisions increase the circumference of the peripheral cornea as they relax tissue around the circumference, transverse incisions, if placed parallel to the limbus and concentric to the center of the visual axis, relax only the meridian in which they are placed and do not increase the corneal circumference. If there is no increase in the circumference of the cornea, a phenomenon called "coupling" occurs. Coupling is the ability of incisions that relax and flatten the steeper meridian to steepen the flatter meridian 90° away (Figure 1-7). The coupling effect of transverse incisions is offset or reduced by added radial incisions or transverse incisions which are so long they become semi-radial.

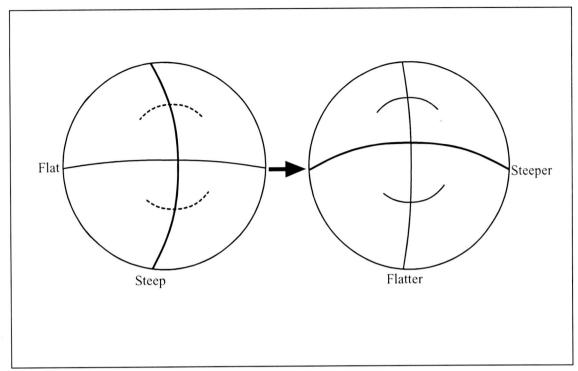

Figure 1-7. Coupling.

The Inverse Arc Incision

All straight lines on spherical surfaces are actually curved (Figure 1-8). Straight transverse incisions are actually inverse arcs and therefore semi-radial. The longer the incision the more radial it becomes (Figure 1-9), reducing any potential coupling.

Taking the concept of arcuate incisions a step further, it can be demonstrated that an exaggerated inverse arc (Figure 1-10) can flatten the steep meridian and at the same time increase the peripheral circumference, reducing myopia. This incision has its greatest use in cases of myopic astigmatism in which reduction of the myopic spherical equivalent, otherwise produced by arcuate incisions, is desired without having to place additional radial incisions. You can reduce the induced myopic spherical equivalent by one-half the amount of the cylinder corrected by using inverse arc incisions (Figure 1-10). The fact that the inverse arc incision does indeed flatten the steep central corneal meridian further refutes the "hinge theory" of meridional flattening.

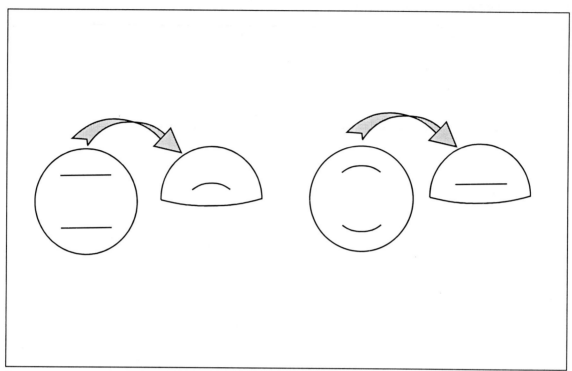

Figure 1-8. Lines on a spherical surface appear straight or curved depending on perspective.

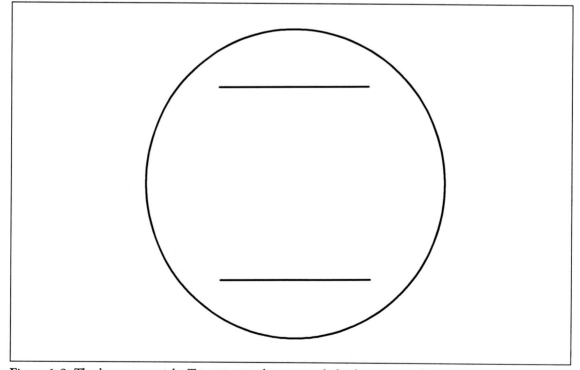

Figure 1-9. The longer a straight T-incision is, the more radial it becomes, reducing coupling.

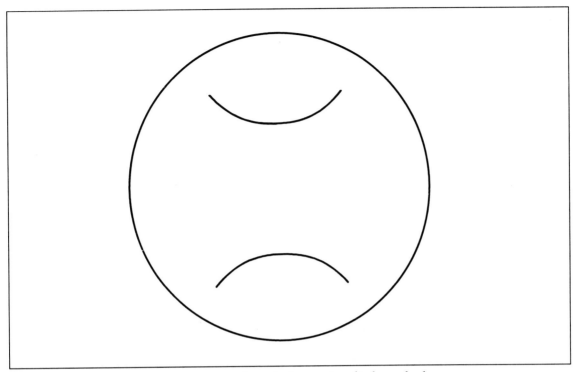

Figure 1-10. An inverse arcuate incision reduces both myopic cylinder and sphere.

Summary

Incisional refractive surgery is becoming a more common method of treating astigmatic errors, whether idiopathic or iatrogenic. Improved diagnostic and surgical equipment, as well as a better understanding of the physiology of the incisions has made the procedure more predictable and effective. The proper techniques of corneal relaxing incisions (astigmatic keratotomy) are easy to learn, and easily performed.

References

1. Fyodorov SN, Ivashina AI, Klimova TL, Kolmanoskii SA (eds): Surgery for anomalies in ocular refraction: a collection of scientific works. The Moscow Research Institute for Ocular Microsurgery, Ministry of Health, RSFSR, 1981.
2. Bores LD, Myers W, Cowden J: Radial Keratotomy: an analysis of the American experience. *Ann Ophthalmol* 13:941-8, 1981.

2

Astigmatic Keratotomy in the Refractive Patient: The ARC-T Study

R. Bruce Grene, MD
Richard L. Lindstrom, MD

The Development of Astigmatic Keratotomy

Astigmatic keratotomy has developed along two historical paths (Figure 2-1). The first path is through the work of traditional corneal surgeons and focuses primarily upon the reduction of postoperative and post-traumatic astigmatism. The combination of relaxing incisions to flatten the steeper meridian, and wedge resections to steepen a flatter meridian, has evolved over a century of work. Initial reports by Schiotz[1] and Bates[2] described the application of perforating astigmatic keratotomy to reduce postkeratoplasty astigmatism. In these cases, as in much of the work that followed, patients had high levels of postoperative astigmatism. More contemporary work can be found in the writings of Troutman.[3] Today, many innovations in the fields of both keratoplasty and cataract surgery prevent high postoperative astigmatism. Nonetheless, we owe many of our modern surgical options for patients with naturally occurring astigmatism to the pioneering work of corneal transplant surgeons.

The second path of development of astigmatic keratotomy was in the field of refractive surgery. The historical difference from traditional corneal surgery is the use of these techniques for patients with naturally occurring astigmatism. This path, too, can trace its origins to work carried out a century ago. In 1895, Faber published a paper about a young man who wished to pursue a

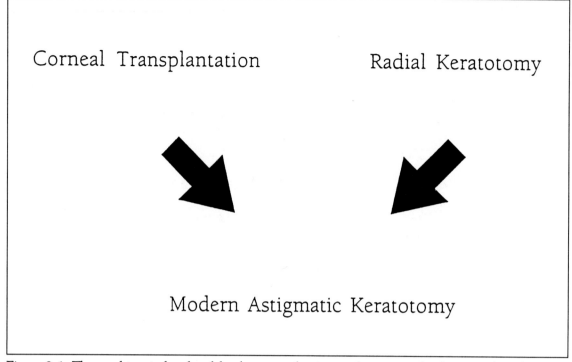

Figure 2-1. The two historical paths of development of astigmatic keratotomy leading to today's dominant schools of approach.

career in the Royal Military Academy and sought improvement of his 20/60 uncorrected visual acuity.[4] Faber used a perforating anterior transverse incision to reduce the 19-year-old's naturally occurring astigmatism. Faber reports a postoperative uncorrected visual acuity of 20/25 allowing the patient to pursue this career path. Two characteristics of this early case helped distinguish it from the traditional cases undertaken by corneal surgeons. The patient had only 1.5 D of pre-existing astigmatism, and he was motivated by a goal of functional necessity. The traditional corneal community would have viewed 1.5 D of regular corneal astigmatism as a marvelous end point and would have been hard pressed to understand the necessity for surgical intervention.

Pioneering work in the field of astigmatic keratotomy can be traced to two giants in the field of refractive surgery: Tsutomu Sato[5] and S. N. Fyodorov.[6] Although well known for their work in developing radial keratotomy, both surgeons contributed to our early understanding of astigmatic keratotomy. Today, radial keratotomy remains the driving force for increased adoption. of astigmatic keratotomy to reduce naturally occurring astigmatism. Astigmatic keratotomy has benefited from the creation of dramatically improved diamond blades and knives, markers, and pachymeters developed by radial keratotomy surgeons.

Modern Schools of Astigmatic Keratotomy

Although the historical divisions between traditional cornea specialists and refractive surgeons were at times rancorous, both groups deserve recognition for parenting modern astigmatic keratotomy. Today's modern schools are led by hybrid surgeons with training in both corneal and refractive surgery. These contemporary leaders have drawn from the best of both schools to help create our modern approach to astigmatic keratotomy. Three modern schools of astigmatic keratotomy are represented by Lee T. Nordan, Richard L. Lindstrom, and Spencer P. Thornton. All three utilize common basic principals of astigmatic keratotomy, but in markedly varied combinations. A brief overview of these three schools illustrates the current dominant approaches to astigmatic keratotomy.

Nordan School

Nordan utilizes three strengths of straight transverse keratotomy to reduce from 1 to 4 D of regular corneal astigmatism.[7] Both his surgical approach and nomogram are the simplest of the three schools (Figure 2-2). Nordan's approach utilizes a single optical zone of 7 mm, a goal for achieved incision depth of 80 to 90%, and assumes a coupling ratio of 2:1 (flattening over steepening). No age factor is utilized.

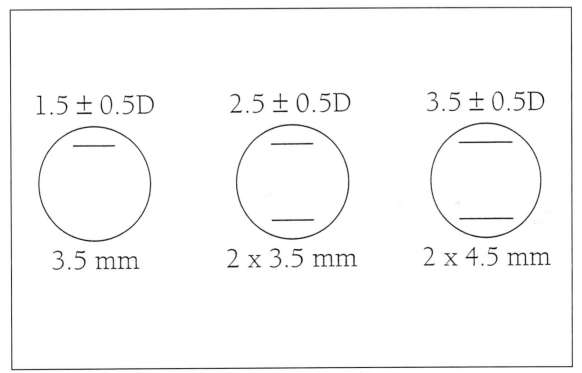

Figure 2-2. Nordan nomogram—Utilizing a single optical zone of 7 mm.

Lindstrom School

Lindstrom's approach to astigmatic keratotomy was the basis for the design of the ARC-T study.[8] Similar to Nordan's approach, a 7-mm optical zone is utilized. A 1.5 coupling ratio was described by Lindstrom and Duffy.[9] Lindstrom's approach has a strong age factor generated by the formula used to create the surgical nomogram (Figure 2-3). The use of arcuate incisions is derived from the work of Merlin.[10] The ARC-T approach corrects from 1 to 7.5 D, depending upon patient age.

Thornton School

Thornton's approach is well described in Chapters 1 and 3. Similarities to Nordan and Lindstrom can be found in the use of both straight T and arcuate transverse incisions. Thornton relies on the use of multiple T-incisions and, accordingly, the use of multiple optical zones. An age factor allows for correction of up to 6 D of regular corneal astigmatism. Thornton assumes a coupling ratio of 1:1.

Basic Principles of Astigmatism

The three schools of astigmatic keratotomy of Nordan, Lindstrom, and Thornton all utilize commonly shared variables in varied combination. Before considering the basic principles of astigmatic keratotomy, it is important to recognize that the description of astigmatism itself varies among leaders in astigmatism surgery. It is essential that our surgical approach be tied to a sound understanding of the optics of astigmatism.

The refractive surgeon must clearly understand and manage three forms of astigmatism; regular, macro irregular, and micro irregular.[11]

Regular Astigmatism

The most common astigmatism, with which all ophthalmologists are familiar, is regular corneal astigmatism. Regular astigmatism is a vector having both magnitude and direction. This astigmatism is correctable with a sphero-cylindrical lens and is the target of surgical reduction by astigmatic keratotomy. We measure regular astigmatism by refraction, keratometry and computerized topography.

Macro Irregular Astigmatism

Two forms of irregular astigmatism must be analyzed in every preoperative and postoperative case. Macro irregular astigmatism refers to regional variations in corneal refracting power. Macro irregular astigmatism is most readily identified by computerized topography (Figure 2-4). In these cases, it is obvious that no two hemimeridians describe the same corneal curvature. Common

	Surgical option				
	2 X 30°		2 X 45°		
AGE	1 X 45°	1 X 60°	1 X 90°	2 X 60°	2 X 90°
20	0.80	1.20	1.60	2.40	3.20
21	0.82	1.23	1.64	2.46	3.28
22	0.84	1.26	1.68	2.52	3.36
23	0.86	1.29	1.72	2.58	3.44
24	0.88	1.32	1.76	2.64	3.52
25	0.90	1.35	1.80	2.70	3.60
26	0.92	1.38	1.84	2.76	3.68
27	0.94	1.41	1.88	2.82	3.76
28	0.96	1.44	1.92	2.88	3.84
29	0.98	1.47	1.96	2.94	3.92
30	1.00	1.50	2.00	3.00	4.00
31	1.02	1.53	2.04	3.06	4.08
32	1.04	1.56	2.08	3.12	4.16
33	1.06	1.59	2.12	3.18	4.24
34	1.08	1.62	2.16	3.24	4.32
35	1.10	1.65	2.20	3.30	4.40
36	1.12	1.68	2.24	3.36	4.48
37	1.14	1.71	2.28	3.42	4.56
38	1.16	1.74	2.32	3.48	4.64
39	1.18	1.77	2.36	3.54	4.72
40	1.20	1.80	2.40	3.60	4.80
41	1.22	1.83	2.44	3.66	4.88
42	1.24	1.86	2.48	3.72	4.96
43	1.26	1.89	2.52	3.78	5.04
44	1.28	1.92	2.56	3.84	5.12
45	1.30	1.95	2.60	3.90	5.20
46	1.32	1.98	2.64	3.96	5.28
47	1.34	2.01	2.68	4.02	5.36
48	1.36	2.04	2.72	4.08	5.44
49	1.38	2.07	2.76	4.14	5.52
50	1.40	2.10	2.80	4.20	5.60
51	1.42	2.13	2.84	4.26	5.68
52	1.44	2.16	2.88	4.32	5.76
53	1.46	2.19	2.92	4.38	5.84
54	1.48	2.22	2.96	4.44	5.92
55	1.50	2.25	3.00	4.50	6.00
56	1.52	2.28	3.04	4.56	6.08
57	1.54	2.31	3.08	4.62	6.16
58	1.56	2.34	3.12	4.68	6.24
59	1.58	2.37	3.16	4.74	6.32
60	1.60	2.40	3.20	4.80	6.40
61	1.62	2.43	3.24	4.86	6.48
62	1.64	2.46	3.28	4.92	6.56
63	1.66	2.49	3.32	4.98	6.64
64	1.68	2.52	3.36	5.04	6.72
65	1.70	2.55	3.40	5.10	6.80
66	1.72	2.58	3.44	5.16	6.88
67	1.74	2.61	3.48	5.22	6.96
68	1.76	2.64	3.52	5.28	7.04
69	1.78	2.67	3.56	5.34	7.12
70	1.80	2.70	3.60	5.40	7.20
71	1.82	2.73	3.64	5.46	7.28
72	1.84	2.76	3.68	5.52	7.36
73	1.86	2.79	3.72	5.58	7.44
74	1.88	2.82	3.76	5.64	7.52
75	1.90	2.85	3.80	5.70	7.60
AGE	1 X 45°	1 X 60°	1 X 90°	2 X 60°	2 X 90°
	2 X 30°		2 X 45°		

Figure 2-3. The ARC-T nomogram based on Lindstrom's formula. The incision option that most closely corrected the total refractive astigmatism was selected.

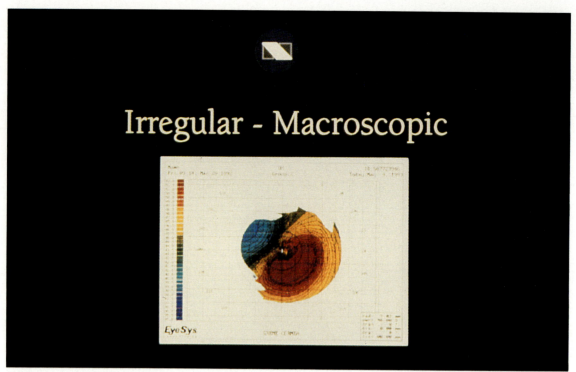

Figure 2-4. Computed topography image demonstrating macro irregular astigmatism.

clinical examples include keratoconus, post keratoplasty, and wound slippage after cataract surgery. Macro irregular astigmatism can be addressed by astigmatic keratotomy, but is more unpredictable in its response to surgery than is regular astigmatism.

Micro Irregular Astigmatism

Micro irregular astigmatism is one of the most powerful diagnostic findings in the preoperative and postoperative management of astigmatism. Micro irregular astigmatism refers to small irregular variations in corneal power. Common clinical entities exhibiting micro irregular astigmatism include keratoconus, SPK, corneal scarring, and the rippling of the anterior corneal surface caused by radial and astigmatic keratotomy incisions. Micro irregular astigmatism is best diagnosed by noting the irregular mires on manual keratometry (Figure 2-5). Difficulty in superimposition of these mires can be graded from 1+ to 4+ in severity. Micro irregular astigmatism is masked by current corneal topography power maps.

The critical importance of this form of astigmatism stems from a number of associated phenomena. Patients with micro irregular astigmatism, despite being capable of 20/20 best-corrected or uncorrected vision, can be profoundly symptomatic from ghosting, which can result in the co-existence of acceptable Snellen acuity and an unhappy, dissatisfied, symptomatic patient.

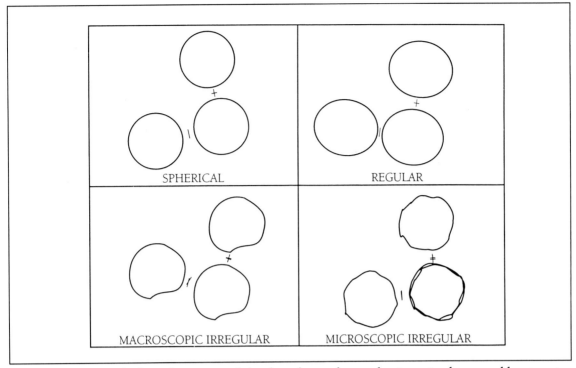

Figure 2-5. Images of spherical corneas and the three forms of corneal astigmatism by manual keratometry.

Additionally, micro irregular astigmatism exaggerates refractive hyperopia and astigmatism.[11,12] Micro irregular astigmatism also helps indicate the presence of wound gape or edema. Detection of residual micro irregular astigmatism is critical to the timing of re-operations for residual regular astigmatism. Patient should have 1+ or less irregular astigmatism prior to placement of additional corneal incisions (enhancement).

Regular Corneal Astigmatism

Collection of Data

The collection of accurate data demands that both the magnitude and axis of the astigmatism be measured accurately. Additionally, one must obtain both keratometric and refractive measures of astigmatism. In general, automated keratometry and automated refraction are unsuitable for preoperative and postoperative measurement of regular corneal astigmatism in patients undergoing astigmatic keratotomy.

Analysis of Data

Even if one is diligent in collecting accurate measurements of both the magnitude and axis of astigmatism, the problem of analyzing the effect of astigmatic keratotomy remains. Four methods for describing the effect of astigmatic keratotomy exist.

The most commonly used approach utilizes the absolute value of the magnitude of either refractive or keratometric cylinder. Although this measurement is easy to obtain and represent, it ignores the effect of over and undercorrection as determined by axis shift. The 3 D astigmat with 1 D of residual astigmatism could have undergone a 2 D effect of surgery with 1 D remaining in the preoperative axis or a 4 D surgical effect with 1 D 90° away from the preoperative axis.

The problem of defining overcorrection is addressed in part by comparing the absolute magnitude of residual refractive or keratometric cylinder with a description of the axis shift induced by surgery. The law of cosines determines the point of overcorrection, ranging from 30-45° depending upon the residual magnitude of astigmatism.[13]

The vector resultant of surgery can be analyzed in the intended meridian of effect. This vector shows the amount of surgical effect in the axis of surgery.[14] Vector analysis has been used with greater frequency in recent publications. Five forms of vector analysis exist in the literature. A brief summary of each form follows:

1. Cravy defined a method of analyzing post cataract extraction astigmatism "...based upon the dynamics of change in curvature of the cornea as determined by keratometry and has no bearing upon refraction, optical lenses, or optical cylinders."[15] Cravy's results are based upon the addition of the changes from the preoperative rectangular coordinate X and Y axis components to the postoperative components—in effect, two legs of a triangle. Vector analysis returns the hypotenuse formed by that triangle.

   Cravy does offer a vector solution in his formulae. However, he has chosen to not use double angle translation to convert the 180° world of visual optics to the 360° world of trigonometry. In that respect, Cravy's vector results differ significantly from the other trigonometric methods.

2. Naylor offered a method of determining the change in astigmatism utilizing the law of cosines.[16] Surgically induced astigmatism, the amount of correction incised in the cornea at the precise axis and length determined by preoperative visual criteria, is represented as a vector. This vector is extrapolated from the geometric relationship of preoperative vector to postoperative vector. The law of cosines adjusts the magnitude of this relationship by adding a trigonometric component to the Pythagorean Theorem (which applies only to right triangles), to account for any angular variations between the two vectors of less than, or greater than, 90°.

   Naylor also provides a solution for the angular component of surgically induced astigmatism. It is this angular component, or more precisely it is calculating this angular component, that generates the multitude of vector analysis methods published over the years. The difficulty arises by the cyclic nature of trigonometric functions. With the exception of the tangent and cotangent functions (and their derivatives), whose periods are asymptomatically bound to $\pi(180°)$, and all angles that are multiples of $\pi/2$ (90°), all trig functions have two angles for each answer. It is determining which angle to use that differentiates the methods. Naylor chose to construct a physical table to graphically provide the correct solution without calculation.

3. Russell, et al. "...developed a new method of calculating astigmatic change that is unique because it is derived from a linear rather than from a trigonometric scale."[17] Russell's formulae alter the magnitude of the surgically induced astigmatic vector by an amount determined by the angular change from preoperative vector to postoperative vector. That amount is a percentage of the change for a maximal shift of 90°. In essence, it is the ratio of the difference between the

two vectors' angular components divided by 90°, multiplied by the difference between the absolute values of the difference between the two vectors' magnitude and the addition of the vectors' magnitude, added to the absolute value of the difference between the vectors magnitudes. It should be noted that though the individual elements used in calculation are vectoral components, there is no provision for determining the angular component for the solution magnitude.

4. The formula developed by Holladay, et al. was initially created to "...address some of the inconsistencies in Cravy's formula."[18] This procedure is based upon a modification of the law of cosines method for solving obliquely crossed cylinders. Similar to Naylor's formulae, trigonometric methodology is used to arrive at the magnitude of the surgically induced astigmatism. The resultant numbers, in fact, are identical to Naylor's.

   The axis of the surgically induced astigmatic vector, as with Naylor's formulae, is the sticking point with this procedure. The angular solution of Holladay's formula, though fundamentally sound, does not provide for the possibility of functions returning the incorrect angle.

   Holladay's strengths include the careful explanations, the generous documentation, instructions on plotting and analyzing data generated by the calculations, and the ability to analyze coupling between the two meridians.

5. A recent addition to the study of vector analysis, Alpins' formula,[19] is based on a rectangular coordinate evaluation of vectoral components. In addition to the surgically induced astigmatic vector, this procedure introduces additional vectors as evaluatory aids. TIA (Target Induced Astigmatism) is the vectoral difference between preoperative astigmatism and targeted astigmatism (in most cases—0 magnitude). The difference vector is, literally, the difference between targeted astigmatism and achieved (postoperative) astigmatism. The assumption here is that by using the variables above "...we can calculate the principle components by which an operation fails to achieve its goals, as well as other components that assist in comparative analysis of astigmatism surgery."

   Alpins' method generates the same values for surgically induced astigmatic magnitude as do Naylor's and Holladay's formulae. Additionally, Alpins' method takes into account the cyclic nature of trigonometric functions, and with a modicum of change (adding a very small amount, 0.0000000001, to the X and Y components of the Targeted Induced Astigmatism) to account for a division by zero error when using targeted astigmatism of zero, Alpins' method generates the correct angular component.

Basic Principles of Astigmatic Keratotomy

Major Variables

The major variables upon which the surgical effect of astigmatic keratotomy is based are well known. The application of these variables make up the ingredients of each school of surgical approach. The golf swings of Palmer, Nicklaus and Watson all look different, yet each relies on common principles configured in different styles. Similarly, Nordan, Lindstrom and Thornton each configure common variables of astigmatic keratotomy differently.

Incision length is a major variable. In general, the longer the incision the greater the effect, all other variables equal. Longer incisions are associated with greater coupling.[7,20] The limit of incision length is controversial, but investigators agree that an upper limit exists beyond which paradoxical flattening of the steeper meridian occurs.

Incision depth is another significant variable. It is generally agreed that AK is less exquisitely sensitive to achieved incision depth than RK. Most surgical approaches recommend an achieved incision depth from 80 to 90%. Perforating incisions are discouraged due to their associated risk of endophthalmitis. Unlike RK microperforations, AK perforations are much less likely to be self-sealing.

The optimal optical zone for astigmatic keratotomy is a subject of great debate. It is generally understood that smaller optical zones are associated with greater surgical effect upon the regular astigmatism. Similarly, this increased effect is associated with increasing micro irregular astigmatism as AK incisions approach the patient's visual axis. This interplay between the increasing power of smaller optical zones and the unwanted increase in micro irregular astigmatism forces surgeons to choose a point of balance between the desired reduction of regular astigmatism and the undesired increase in micro irregular astigmatism.

The optimal configuration for astigmatic keratotomy incisions remains the subject of intense clinical research. The recent ARC-T study analyzed arcuate incisions in 159 eyes and will be presented in detail in this chapter.[8] A recently completed analysis of 100 arcuate transverse incisions versus 100 straight transverse incisions was done in an effort to determine the preferred incision configuration for AK.[21] Chevron and inverse arcuate incisions complete the menu of possible AK configurations.

The optimal number of incisions remains, once again, the subject of debate. Increasing numbers of incisions increase the complexity of the surgical procedure but offers the advantage of distributing corneal bending over multiple incisions. This strategy has the potential of reducing the risk of incision gape and its associated complications of overcorrection and permanent irregular astigmatism.

Limits of AK

Each school of approach to astigmatic keratotomy is faced with the same limits of incisional astigmatic correction. These limits must be respected to avoid unwanted side effects and complications for our patients.

Any reasonable application of the major variables listed above is limited in power, making AK best suited for low and moderate amounts of astigmatism. The exact upper range varies from 4 to 7 D. Beyond this level the limiting factors listed below begin to diminish the safety of AK.

Irregular astigmatism occurs as a result of excessive corneal bending or through the placement of transverse incisions too close to the visual axis. Irregular astigmatism creates image degradation, experienced as ghosting by the patient.

The phenomenon of wound gape limits the amount of astigmatic keratotomy reasonably attempted. Wound gape is associated with irregular astigmatism as well as overcorrection of regular astigmatism. Although generally ameliorated by suturing the gaped incision, wound gape remains a common complication of AK.

Corneal stability begins to be affected at the upper limits of astigmatic keratotomy. Although AK is less sensitive to visual fluctuation than RK, astigmatic keratotomy is nonetheless a corneal weakening surgery with potential risk of excessive destabilization of the cornea. It is not known whether AK creates less instability than RK, whether patients are less aware of fluctuating cylinder, or if fluctuation in cylinder is harder to measure than changes in sphere.

ARC-T Study

Objectives

In an effort to better understand astigmatic keratotomy, a group of nine surgeons performed arcuate transverse keratotomy on 159 eyes. Objectives included the determination of the effect of arcuate transverse incisions on corneal and refractive astigmatism. The study assessed the reliability of postoperative manual keratometry by comparison to calculated values. The predictability of the surgical nomogram was evaluated. Finally, complications and side effects associated with astigmatic keratotomy are reported.

Methods

Astigmatic keratotomy was performed on 159 eyes using arcuate incisions and a 7-mm optical zone. All nine surgeons used the same instrumentation, surgical technique, and nomogram.

Inclusion criteria required that patients be at least 18 years of age with 1 to 6 D of naturally occurring astigmatism. The nomogram provided predictions for seven surgical options (Figure 2-6). Both single arcuate incisions of 45°, 60° or 90° in length and paired incisions of 30°, 45°, 60° or 90° in length used a 7-mm optical zone (Figure 2-7). The surgeons were advised to choose the surgical plan that most closely corrected the total refractive cylinder without overcorrecting. The ARC-T nomogram includes an age factor.

Results

Vector analysis was utilized to determine the net effect of astigmatic keratotomy on refractive and corneal astigmatism. The patients ranged from 18 to 66 years of age with a mean of 39.5 years. The population was 67% female and 33% male. The mean value for preoperative refractive cylinder was 2.8 D (Table 2-1). Only 10% of the population had against-the-rule astigmatism. At one month, 43% of cases had residual refractive astigmatism within 0.50 D of plano. Residual astigmatism of 1 D or less was measured in 71% of the cases. The rate of overcorrection greater than 1 D was 6% (Table 2-2). Complications were infrequent and minimal in severity.

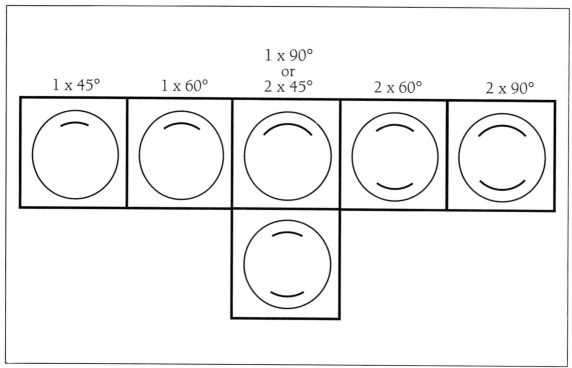

Figure 2-6. Surgical options referred to by the ARC-T nomogram.

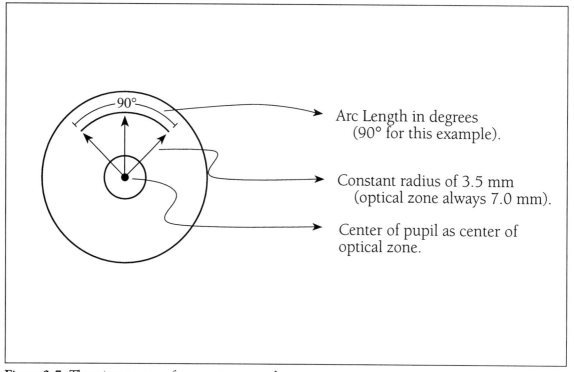

Figure 2-7. The trigonometry of arcuate transverse keratotomy.

Table 2-1.

Preoperative Demographics	N	Mean	SD	Median	Min	Max
Age: All	159	39.47	9.69	38	18	66
Age: Male (33%)	53	42.87	9.93	42	20	66
Age: Female (67%)	106	37.76	9.15	37	18	64
Refractive astigmatism: All	159	2.78	1.22	2.50	1.00	6.50
Refractive astigmatism: Male	53	2.96	1.35	2.50	1.25	6.50
Refractive astigmatism: Female	106	2.67	1.14	2.50	1.00	6.25
Keratometric astigmatism	159	2.68	1.13	2.50	0.50	6.00
Lenticular Astigmatism	159	0.82	0.49	0.75	0.00	2.63

Table 2-1. Statistical evaluation of preoperative information. Astigmatism is measured in diopters.

Table 2-2.
Change in refractive astigmatism derived through the
"Holladay, Cravy, Koch" method of vector analysis

N = 159	±0.50 D		±1.00 D	
	No.	%	No.	%
Within range	69	43	113	71
Overcorrection	20	13	10	6
Undercorrection	70	44	36	23

Conclusion

Arcuate keratotomy reduces corneal and refractive astigmatism. Although serious complications were infrequent, irregular astigmatism was a common sequela of surgery. A follow-up analysis of six month results is underway to assess the stability of these results and the predictability of the ARC-T nomogram.

Issues in Astigmatic Keratotomy

Astigmatic keratotomy is clearly a viable option for the symptomatic astigmat. Improvements in both instrumentation and technique offer the patient a surgical option that is generally both safe and effective. It is true that the predictability of astigmatic keratotomy remains unacceptable, but there is great reason for optimism that the next decade will bring dramatic improvement in predictability of astigmatic keratotomy. Several important issues face refractive surgeons challenged with improving astigmatic keratotomy.

Alternatives

Laser

The first challenge to improving astigmatic surgery is to recognize alternatives to incisional keratotomy. Excimer laser is currently in clinical trials to develop a non-incisional means of flattening the steeper corneal meridian. In contrast to astigmatic keratotomy, current laser techniques also flatten the flatter meridian. This "reverse coupling" phenomenon is important to consider in the selection of a surgical approach. The patient who is +1.00 -2.00 preoperatively is a much better candidate for astigmatic keratotomy. A 2:1 coupling ratio offers the potential of a plano postoperative result. Conversely, the patient that is -1.00 -2.00 preoperatively should be considered for excimer laser photoastigmatic keratectomy (see Chapter 4). The simultaneous flattening of both steep and flatter meridians with 2 to 1 emphasis of effect in the steeper meridian would also bring this patient to plano.

Range

One challenge facing refractive surgeons today is to better define the appropriate range of astigmatic keratotomy. The most frequent side effect of our surgeries is wound gape with overcorrection of regular astigmatism or creation of permanent micro irregular astigmatism. The current literature with adequate series of patients describes populations with less than 2 D mean preoperative cylinder (Thornton 1.50 D, Neumann 1.32 D).[22,23] Even the ARC-T study population had only 2.8 D mean preoperative cylinder. A significant question exists regarding the appropriate surgical technique for the reduction of 4 to 7 D of naturally occurring regular corneal astigmatism.

Instrumentation

The last decade's improvement of instrumentation for astigmatic keratotomy has markedly improved surgical technique. Nonetheless, there is a critical need for improved methods of identifying and marking at surgery the exact meridian of steepest corneal curvature. Accurate treatment at the steep corneal meridian is even more critical in laser photoastigmatic keratectomy.

Configuration

Another active issue in astigmatic keratotomy research is that of incision configuration. The effect of straight, arcuate, or inverse arcuate incisions upon the power, predictability, and side effects of astigmatic keratotomy bears further study. The use of case reports should be replaced by the collection of larger series of procedures. These studies demand critical measurement of the magnitude and axis of both refractive and keratometric astigmatism, as well as vector analysis of the results of surgery.

Optical Zone

The appropriate optical zone for astigmatic keratotomy, as in radial keratotomy, is dependent upon a broader recognition of the insidious influence of micro irregular astigmatism. So long as refractive surgeons measure only uncorrected vision as the standard of surgical success, we will continue to create surgical techniques that lead to significant ghosting and visual disability for our patients. Exciting new computerized techniques are being developed to accurately map the distribution of micro irregular astigmatism. For now, all refractive surgeons should examine the clarity of the mires on manual keratometry. This simple diagnostic test offers tremendous reward in better understanding the optical side effects of our refractive surgical procedures, as well as a means of following wound healing post AK.

Re-operation

Improved strategies for dealing with re-operation for both under and overcorrection are needed. As astigmatic keratotomy has evolved it becomes clear that, much like radial keratotomy, it is a surgical procedure that frequently requires multiple procedures. Many questions surround the issue of astigmatic keratotomy enhancement. What is the desired goal of astigmatic keratotomy? What is more important to our patient's vision—residual magnitude or postoperative axis? What is the most effective means of enhancing undercorrected regular corneal astigmatism—additional incisions, lengthening of incisions, deepening of incisions, or a combination of these techniques? What are the most effective means of dealing with overcorrection of astigmatic keratotomy? What sutures are best tolerated and how long should they remain in place? Do patients with and without significant wound gape respond differently to suture compression?

Summary

The field of astigmatism surgery is entering its second century.[24] Despite the many triumphs of improved technique and technology, much remains to be learned about the effect of astigmatic keratotomy. The synergistic cooperation of traditional corneal transplant surgeons and radial keratotomy specialists gives astigmatic surgery the balance of careful analysis and clinical practicality it needs to become an integral part of all anterior segment surgeons' armamentarium.

References

1. Schiotz HA: Ein Fall von hochgradigem Hornhautastigmatismus nach Staarextraction. Besserung auf operativem Wege. *Archiv fur Augenheilkunde* 15:178-181, 1885.

2. Bates WH: A suggestion of an operation to correct astigmatism. *Arch Ophthalmol* 23:9-19, 1894.

3. Troutman RC: *Microsurgery of the Anterior Segment of the Eye.* St. Louis, MO, CV Mosby Co, p. 286, 1987.

4. Faber E: Operative Behandeling van Astigmatisme. *Nederl Tijdschr V Geneesk* 2:495-496, 1985.

5. Sato T: The cause and prevention of myopia. *Kosei no Nippon Sha,* 1944.

6. Fyodorov SN, Durner VV: Surgical correction of complicated myopic astigmatism by means of dissection of circular ligament of cornea. *Ann Ophthalmol* 13:115-118, 1981.

7. Nordan LT, Hofbauer JD: Astigmatism: concepts and surgical approach - irregular astigmatism. In: Nordan LT, Maxwell WA, Davison JA, eds, *The Surgical Rehabilitation of Vision.* New York, NY, Gower Medical Publishing, 1992.

8. Grene RB, Kenyon KR, Durrie DS, et al: Astigmatism reduction clinical trial: a multi-center prospective evaluation of the surgical results of arcuate keratotomy for the reduction of astigmatism. 1993 (in press).

9. Duffey RJ, Jain VN, Tchah H, Hoffman RF, Lindstrom RL: Paired arcuate keratotomy: a surgical approach to mixed and myopic astigmatism. *Arch Ophthalmol* 106:1130-5, 1988.

10. Merlin U: Curved keratotomy procedure for congenital astigmatism. *Journal of Refractive Surgery* 3:92-97, 1987.

11. Grene RB: Astigmatism chapter. In: Roy FH, ed, *Ophthalmic Surgery: Approaches of the Masters.* Philadelphia, PA, Lee & Febiger, in press.

12. Nordan LT, Grene RB: The importance of corneal asphericity and irregular astigmatism in refractive surgery. *Refract Corneal Surg* 6(3);200-4, 1990.

13. Grene RB, Kerr LG: Surgically induced refractive change: evaluation of current methods to calculate change in astigmatism following astigmatic keratotomy. Unpublished.

14. Thornton SP, Sanders DR: Graded nonintersecting transverse incisions for correction of idiopathic astigmatism. *J Cataract Refract Surg* 13(1):27-31, 1987.

15. Cravy TV: Calculation of the change in corneal astigmatism following cataract extraction. *Ophthalmic Surg* 10(1):38-49, 1979.

16. Naylor EJ: Astigmatic difference in refractive errors. *Br J Ophthalmol* 52:422-425, 1968.

17. Russell JT, Koch DD, Gay CA: A new formula to calculate changes in corneal astigmatism. Unpublished.

18. Holladay JT, Cravy TV, Koch DD: Calculating the surgically induced refractive change following ocular surgery. *J Cataract Refract Surg* 18:429-443, 1992.

19. Alpins NA: A new method of analyzing vectors for change in astigmatism. *J Cataract Refract Surg* 19:524-533, 1993.

20. Waring GO, Holladay JT: *Refractive Keratotomy for Myopia and Astigmatism.* St. Louis, MO, Mosby Year Book, Inc., 1992.

21. Grene RB: ARC-T versus straight-T: 100 cases. 1993. Unpublished.

22. Thornton SP: Astigmatic keratotomy: a review of basic concepts with case reports. *J Cataract Refract Surg* 16(4):430-5, 1990.

23. Neumann AC, McCarty GR, Sanders DR, Raanan MG: Refractive evaluation of astigmatic keratotomy procedures. *J Cataract Refract Surg* 15(1)25-31, 1989.

24. Lindstrom RL: Lans Distinguished Refractive Surgery Lecture: The surgical correction of astigmatism: a clinician's perspective. *Refractive & Corneal Surgery* 6:441-454, 1990.

3

Astigmatic Keratotomy in the Cataract Patient

James P. Gills, MD
Robert G. Martin, MD
Spencer P. Thornton, MD, FACS

Introduction

With the safety and efficacy of astigmatic keratotomy well established and the advantages of intraocular lenses long accepted, the aim of the progressive cataract surgeon has become achieving emmetropia in the cataract patient.

The architecture of cataract incisions has been improved to the point that surgically induced astigmatism has been markedly reduced. Cataract incisions have become smaller, inducing less astigmatism, and the use of scleral-pocket three-stage incisions and clear-corneal entry has resulted in essentially astigmatically neutral wounds. In addition, by proper placement of cataract incisions in the steep corneal axis, we have been able to reduce some of the patient's pre-existing astigmatism.

Astigmatic keratotomy is not a difficult procedure to perform, and, as you will see from the discussion which follows, safe, accurate techniques are within the reach of every skilled ophthalmic surgeon.

Astigmatism and Cataract Surgery

When Should Corneal Relaxing Incisions Be Done?

The question now being asked with increasing frequency is, "Should I perform corneal relaxing incisions (CRIs) at the time of cataract surgery or wait several months after surgery?" The answer will depend both on your philosophy and the certainty of your astigmatic-neutral cataract surgery.

On the one hand, the astigmatic effect of cataract surgery—even with small incisions, and in the best of surgical hands—is sometimes not as accurate as the surgeon would desire, and some postoperative corneal curvature changes can surprise you. On the other hand, patients are often reluctant to undergo an additional procedure after the cataract surgery is performed, even if the procedure may substantially improve their uncorrected vision.

Who Should Receive Corneal Relaxing Incisions?

Patient selection depends in large part on the surgeon's personal philosophy toward correcting astigmatism. Surgeons generally will not attempt correction of astigmatism with relaxing incisions below a certain level, but what that minimum level of pre-existing astigmatism is varies from surgeon to surgeon. Today, most surgeons who wish to correct low levels of pre-existing astigmatism will do so with cataract wound management techniques (see Section IV), and reserve relaxing incisions for moderate to high levels of astigmatism.

Many surgeons are also cautious about attempting correction of with-the-rule astigmatism, lest there is an overcorrection and the cylinder ends up against-the-rule postoperatively. Since against-the-rule cylinder is harder for patients to tolerate, many surgeons will deliberately target substantial undercorrection to avoid an axis shift, or not perform relaxing incisions for with-the-rule cylinder unless the astigmatism level is relatively high.

Techniques and Results of Corneal Relaxing Incisions in Cataract Patients

The Martin Approach

Corneal relaxing incisions can be performed with either scleral-tunnel sutureless cataract incisions or clear-corneal cataract incisions. If a scleral-tunnel incision is used, the incision is placed superiorly. If a clear-corneal cataract incision is used, the incision can be placed temporally or at the steep axis of preoperative astigmatism.

Table 3-1.
Martin Nomogram for Arcuate Corneal Relaxing Incisions

Age	Dioptric Effect Per mm of Chord Length
20-29	0.50 D
30-39	0.55 D
40-49	0.65 D
50-59	0.70 D
60-69	0.75 D
70 and up	0.80 D

Table 3-2.
Martin Nomogram for Arcuate Corneal Relaxing Incisions Placed in Same Meridian as Clear-Corneal Sutureless Cataract Incision

Age	Dioptric Effect Per mm of Chord Length
20-29	0.60 D
30-39	0.70 D
40-49	0.80 D
50-59	0.90 D
60-69	0.95 D
70 and up	1.00 D

Table 3-1 outlines the Martin nomogram for corneal relaxing incisions. All CRIs are arcuate. If one pair is used, it is placed at the 7-mm optical zone. Additional pairs at the 8- or 9-mm optical zone provide an additional 50% more effect. The cuts are never less than 1.5 mm in chord length, or more than 3.5 mm in chord length at the 7-mm optical zone. Avoid cuts within the 5-mm optical zone.

Age is a major factor in the effect of the incisions. The incision size for a 20 to 29 year-old patient needs to be about twice the size as for a 70 year-old patient to get the same effect.

If the CRIs are made in the same meridian as a clear-corneal sutureless cataract incision, add approximately 10% more power per mm (Table 3-2). If the CRIs are made at right angles to the sutureless cataract incision, subtract 10% less power per mm.

The primary goal is to reduce against-the-rule astigmatism postoperatively. The surgeon attempts to correct all of the against-the-rule cylinder, because if an overcorrection occurs, the residual cylinder will be with-the-rule. However, great care should be taken to avoid overcorrection of with-the-rule cylinder, to avoid residual against-the-rule cylinder. Thus, with-the-rule cases should be approached more conservatively than against-the-rule cases.

Surgical Technique

The surgical technique for astigmatic keratotomy consists of measuring the central 2 mm of corneal astigmatism using corneal topography. A nomogram is then used to calculate the degrees, or millimeters, of cut at optical zone 7. The plus axis of astigmatism is then confirmed intraoperatively with a corneoscope. The cornea is dried, a 7-mm marker applied and the amount of incision marked with a caliper. Pachymetric measurements are made precisely on the site to be cut.

The technician inspects the blade to make sure it is not dirty or contaminated by protein build-up, improperly aligned, or chipped or damaged. Any of these conditions will markedly decrease the depth of incision and surgical efficacy. The micrometer knife is set at 100% pachymetric depth. A pointed diamond blade or tri-faceted blade is used to cut arcuate incisions. The blade is rolled slightly with the fingers to create an arc. Incisions are always cut perpendicular to the globe, otherwise the incision will shelve and be too shallow. Incisions are cut slowly to avoid macroperforations.

Results

A consecutive cohort of 29 cases receiving a superiorly-placed, scleral-tunnel, sutureless cataract incision and one pair of CRIs, operated upon between January and May, 1993, was analyzed. Data were collected retrospectively through chart review. All cases had two and a half to four month follow-up. The mean age was 69.7 years and 62% were male.

Preoperatively no case had less than 1 D of keratometric cylinder (Figure 3-1). The majority of cases (83%) had 2 D or more. Postoperatively, 28% had less than 1 D of cylinder and 62% had less than 2 D.

Figure 3-2 is a scatterplot of the individual changes in keratometric cylinder from preoperative levels to three months postoperatively. Points falling below the solid line indicate cases with reduced cylinder, while points falling within the dashed lines indicate cases within 0.5 D of preoperative levels. Postoperatively, 72% (21/29) had residual cylinder which was reduced from the preoperative level by over 0.5 D. Two cases had higher levels of cylinder postoperatively, one by about 1 D and one by about 0.5 D.

Vector methods were used to calculate how much cylinder was surgically induced in the axis 90° away from the preoperative steep axis, that is, in the direction which would correct preoperative cylinder. Theoretically, perfect correction occurs when the total surgically induced change to corneal shape is a cylinder vector in the correcting direction and is equal in magnitude to preoperative cylinder. Figure 3-3 is a scatterplot of the amount of cylinder induced in the correcting direction versus preoperative cylinder. Points falling below the equivalency line indicate undercorrected cases and points above the line are overcorrected cases. Overcorrections do result in axis shifts. Points within the dashed lines are cases within 0.5 D of a perfect correction. Three cases were overcorrected by slightly over half a diopter and one case by about 2.5 D, but the majority were either within 0.5 D of attempted correction or were mildly undercorrected.

Figure 3-4 shows the preoperative versus postoperative cylinder axis. For most cases, postoperative cylinder axis is quite close to preoperative. Ten cases with against-the-rule cylinder preoperatively had axis shifts resulting in with-the-rule astigmatism postoperatively. These cases are indicated by triangles on the graph. Eight of these ten cases had decreases in the magnitude of

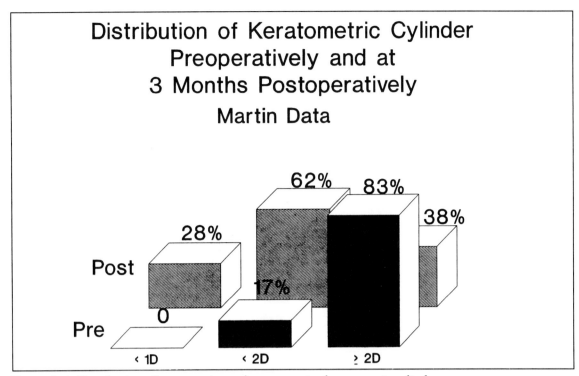

Figure 3-1. Distribution of preoperative and postoperative keratometric cylinder.

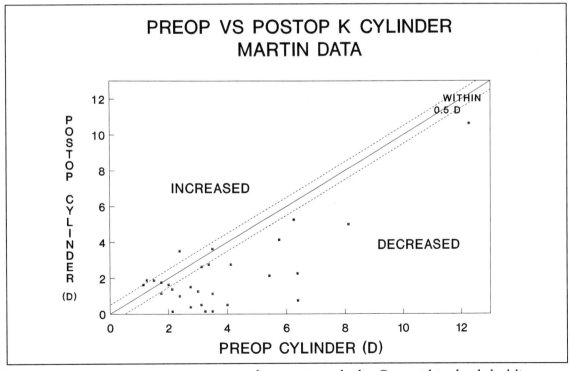

Figure 3-2. Postoperative versus preoperative keratometric cylinder. Cases within the dashed lines were within 0.5 D of preoperative cylinder postoperatively. Cases below the solid line had a decrease in cylinder, while cases above had an increase.

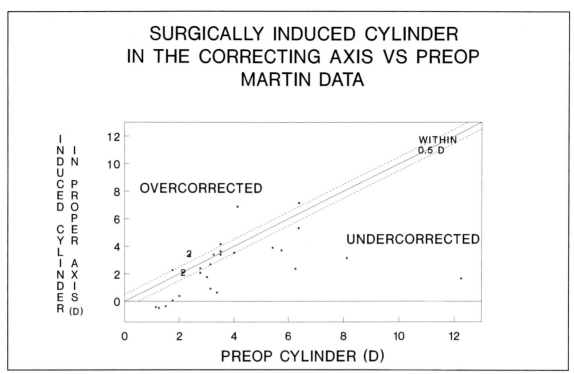

Figure 3-3. Amount of surgically induced cylinder 90° away from the preoperative steep keratometric axis (correcting axis) versus preoperative cylinder. Cases within the dashed lines were within 0.5 D of a perfect correction. Cases below the solid line received a partial correction, while cases above were overcorrected.

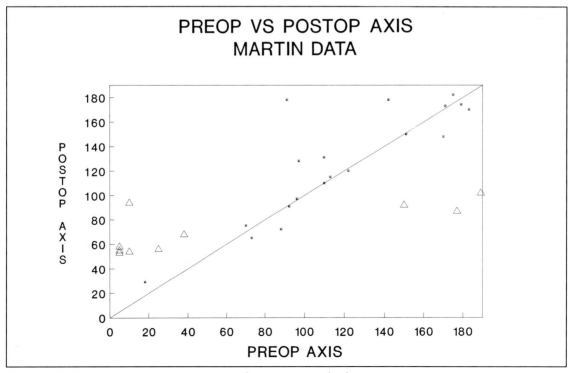

Figure 3-4. Postoperative versus preoperative keratometric cylinder axis.

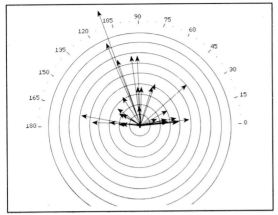

Figure 3-5A. Preoperative cylinder.

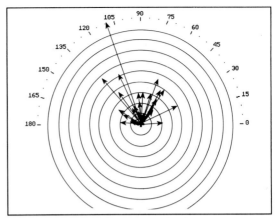

Figure 3-5B. Postoperative cylinder.

Figure 3-5. Vector representation of the Martin series. The length of each arrow represents the magnitude of keratometric cylinder and the direction as indicated by the dial represents the steep cylinder axis for each case. Each concentric circle represents 1 D.

the residual cylinder. One case of with-the-rule cylinder was overcorrected, resulting in postoperative against-the-rule cylinder.

Figure 3-5 illustrates the effect of this surgical procedure on the cohort as a whole. The cylinder vector for each case is represented as a vector arrow, where the length of the vector is the cylinder power, and the direction (as indicated around the dial) is the axis. Figure 3-5A shows the preoperative cylinder and Figure 3-5B shows the postoperative cylinder. The space between each concentric circle represents 1 D. Preoperatively more than half the cases are against-the-rule, and 55% of the cases have more than 3 D of cylinder. Postoperatively there is a decided preponderance of with-the-rule cylinder (72% of cases), and the magnitude of cylinder is greatly reduced in most cases. More than half the cases have 2 D or less cylinder postoperatively, and 72% have 3 D or less. These graphs show that the goals of surgery are generally achieved in the group as a whole: less residual against-the-rule cylinder and a general reduction in cylinder level.

Topographic Evaluation of Superior Sutureless Scleral-Tunnel Cataract Incision with Arcuate CRIs

Figure 3-6 shows the corneal topography of a 79 year-old man who received a 3.2-mm sutureless scleral-tunnel cataract incision and a pair of arcuate relaxing incisions. The temporal incision had a chord length of 2.9 mm while the nasal incision had a chord length of 3.1 mm.

Preoperatively, the patient had 3.25 D of keratometric cylinder. Four months postoperatively the keratometry indicated essentially sphericity. The topographic change image (bottom) indicates that in the meridian of the incision essentially no change has occurred, but that elsewhere in the cornea slight steepening has occurred. The most steepening occurred 90° away from the incisions, where the cornea had previously been flattest. The patient achieved excellent visual acuity, seeing 20/20 uncorrected.

Figure 3-7 illustrates the topography of a 77 year-old man who received a 3.2-mm sutureless scleral-tunnel incision and a pair of CRIs to counteract large with-the-rule astigmatism. Both the

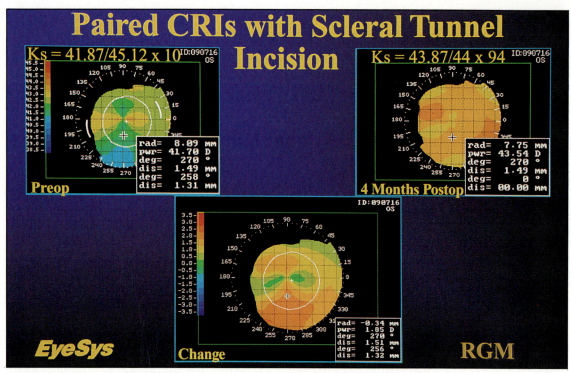

Figure 3-6. Corneal topography of a case receiving a superior scleral-tunnel cataract incision and one pair of relaxing incisions to correct pre-existing against-the-rule astigmatism. Upper left shows preoperative corneal appearance, upper right shows four month postoperative appearance, and bottom shows surgically induced corneal changes.

inferior and superior incision had a chord length of 3 mm. Because the cylinder was with-the-rule, a conservative approach was taken.

Preoperatively, the patient had over 8 D of keratometric cylinder. The topography showed severely asymmetric astigmatism, with the cornea steepest inferiorly. Postoperatively the topography showed the same astigmatic pattern, with a reduction in the steepness. The keratometric cylinder has been reduced by over 3 D, leaving 5 D of residual cylinder. The patient achieved reasonably good visual acuity, seeing 20/40 uncorrected and 20/20 corrected.

The Gills Approach

Cases with less than 0.5 D of astigmatism receive either a standard scleral-tunnel or clear-corneal cataract incision. In cases with 0.5 D, a clear-corneal incision is placed at the steep axis. For cases with 0.75 D to 3 D of cylinder we aim for correcting approximately two-thirds of the preoperative cylinder. This procedure places the sutureless cataract incision as well as a single relaxing incision in the steep meridian. For against-the-rule astigmatism, we use a clear-corneal cataract incision in a temporal location, and for with-the-rule astigmatism we use scleral-tunnel incisions, superiorly.

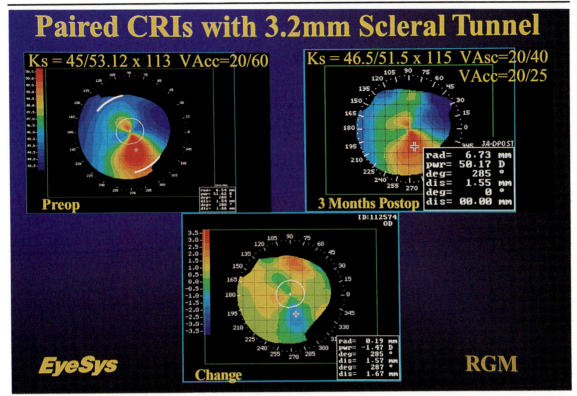

Figure 3-7. Corneal topography of a case receiving a superior scleral-tunnel cataract incision and one pair of relaxing incisions to correct pre-existing with-the-rule astigmatism. Upper left shows preoperative corneal appearance, upper right shows three month postoperative appearance, and bottom shows surgically induced corneal changes. Postoperatively the astigmatic pattern remains the same, but the magnitude has lessened.

The steep meridian is determined by using keratometry, the Terry keratometer, and corneal topography. In addition, the axis is re-measured at surgery with the Terry keratometer to ensure accuracy. The relaxing incision is 2 mm in length for every diopter of preoperative cylinder. We generally place the relaxing incision immediately anterior to the cataract incision. If corneal topography indicates asymmetrical astigmatism, however, we place the relaxing incision where the cornea is steepest.

We previously placed CRIs at the 7-mm optical zone, but now use an 8-mm optical zone. Although with a larger optical zone a larger incision is required to correct the same level of astigmatism, the relaxing incision at this location produces less irregular astigmatism, distortion and glare.

Surgical Technique

The patient is subjected to careful evaluation and consideration with an explanation of all the risks. The patient then has topography and keratometry to determine the amount and axis of the astigmatism. The steep axis is marked with a little cautery burn on the conjunctiva at the steep meridian. The mark is made so it will not wash off and is significant enough to last through multiple doses of betadine. Pachymetry readings are taken to determine incision depth settings.

After the axis has been marked the patient is taken to the operating room. Usually after the cataract procedure, the axis of the steep meridian has a relaxing incision on one side and possibly on two sides if there is over 3.0 to 3.5 D of astigmatism. The cataract incision is usually made in the steep meridian, so with a clear-corneal cataract incision the relaxing incision is usually just anterior, in the 8-mm optical zone (Figure 3-8). If the clear-corneal incision is made temporally and the patient has a very steep nasal meridian, the relaxing incision is performed in the 8-mm optical zone opposite to the cataract incision.

Figures 3-9 through 3-11 show the instruments used in the astigmatic keratotomy procedure. The eye is fixated with the Thornton fixation ring (Storz), and the Thornton arcuate marker (Storz) imprints the cornea to make performing accurate incisions easy. The incisions are made with the Thornton arcuate keratotomy knife (Storz).

The surgeon attempts 100% depth, without perforating into the anterior chamber. The surgeon attempts to deepen the cut approximately 0.1 mm and measure on track if it is close to the area where the clear-corneal incision is because there is increased edema associated with phacoemulsification in that area. A 2-mm incision in the steep meridian, approximately 100% deep, usually relieves approximately 0.8 D of astigmatism. Since slight undercorrection is targeted, a 2.0 mm cut per diopter of astigmatism is made. Incisions over 3.0 mm long create an increased effect. From 3.0 mm to 4.5 mm there is a more variable response, but they can achieve approximately 1.2 to 1.5 D of effect per mm. So, a 4.5-mm incision can achieve 4 or 5 D of effect on some occasions. However, on most occasions a 3.0-mm to 4.0-mm incision will achieve about 1.0 D of effect for every 2 mm of cut.

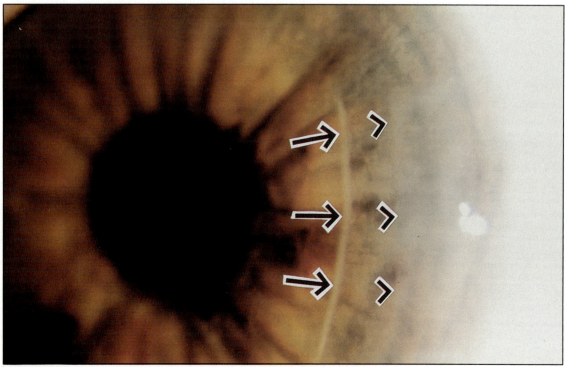

Figure 3-8. Clinical appearance postoperatively of clear-corneal cataract incision (carets) and adjacent CRI (arrows).

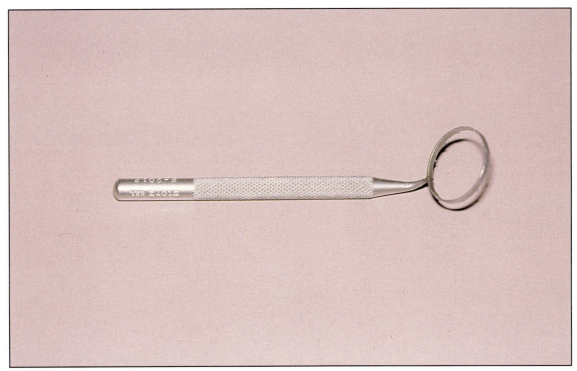

Figure 3-9. Thornton fixation ring.

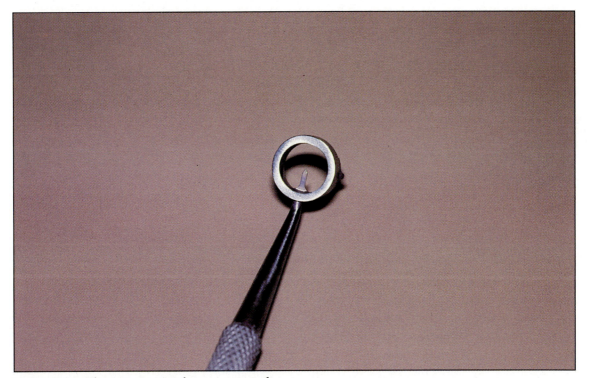

Figure 3-10. Thornton arcuate keratotomy marker.

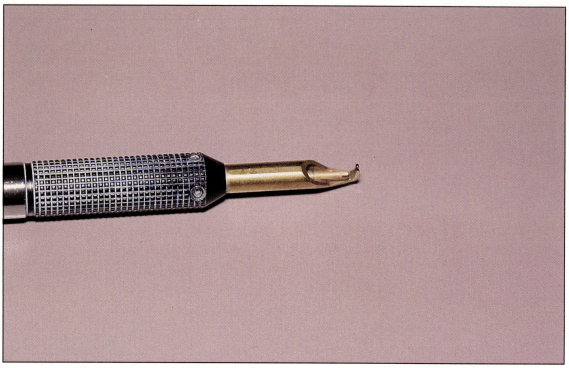

Figure 3-11. Thornton arcuate keratotomy knife.

The eyes are evaluated following the incisions at the time of surgery with the Terry keratometer. The patient can then be re-refracted, sometimes immediately after the cuts, to see what effect the surgery has had. If the preoperative astigmatism is large, perhaps as much as 6.0 to 8.0 D, more surgery can be performed on the same day. Most of the time, however, a second procedure would be performed several weeks later.

Patients always have topical antibiotics applied to the eye. The eye is rarely patched, but occasionally a contact lens is used if there is any abrasion of the epithelium. If the epithelium has been displaced, the surgeon makes an effort to place it back in its original position.

Results

A cohort of 53 cases with against-the-rule astigmatism receiving a temporal clear-corneal incision and a single or pair of CRIs was analyzed. Forty-two of these cases had data between one and three weeks postoperatively and 33 had two to four month data.

Vector analysis methods were used to calculate the surgically induced cylinder. Figure 3-12 demonstrates the attempted axis of surgically induced cylinder, that is, the axis 90° away from the steep axis of preoperative cylinder, versus the actual axis of induced cylinder at the two to four month visit. Points close to the equivalency line indicate well-directed surgical effect. Most of the points are within 10° of the equivalency line, demonstrating excellent accuracy.

We then calculated how much of the induced cylinder was induced in the direction which would correct preoperative cylinder (the attempted axis, or correcting axis). The postoperative

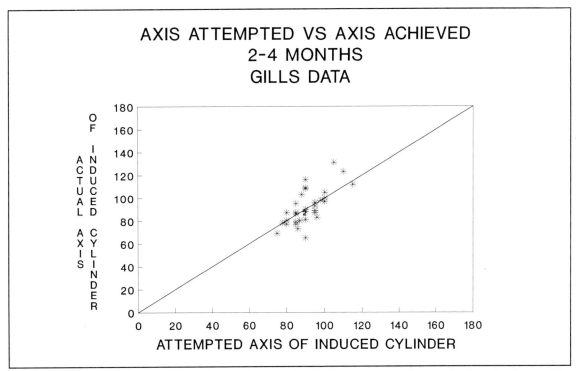

Figure 3-12. Scatterplot of attempted axis of induced cylinder versus actual axis of induced cylinder. The attempted axis is defined as 90° away from the steep preoperative cylinder axis. Points close to the equivalency line indicate good surgical accuracy.

pattern often is overcorrection early with subsequent regression. At the one to three week visit (Figure 3-13A), about half of the cases were within 0.5 D of a spherical correction, while most of the rest were, in fact, overcorrected. By the two to four month visit (Figure 3-13B), the early overcorrections had mostly regressed. Most cases were within 0.5 D of a spherical correction, while eight cases were undercorrected and four cases remained overcorrected. It also appears that cases with larger amounts of preoperative cylinder who received longer incisions achieved greater surgical effect.

Figure 3-14 is a scatterplot of preoperative versus postoperative cylinder without regard to axis at the later postoperative visit. The vast majority of cases showed a reduction of at least 0.5 D in cylinder by this time period, and most had a diopter or more reduction. One case had a negligible (0.25 D) increase in cylinder.

Figures 3-15A and 3-15B demonstrate the preoperative and two to four month postoperative cylinder vectors for the cohort as a whole. The length of the vector represents the cylinder magnitude, while the direction indicated on the dial represents the steep axis. Each concentric circle represents 0.5 D. Preoperatively, all cases in the cohort are against-the-rule. Postoperatively, about 1/4 of the cases are with-the-rule. These figures demonstrate the dramatic reduction in cylinder. Preoperatively, no case has less than 1 D of cylinder, but postoperatively, half the cases have less than 0.5 D, and 82% have 1 D or less.

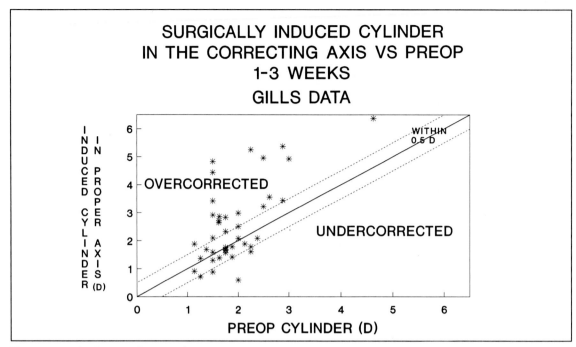

Figure 3-13A. One to three week visit.

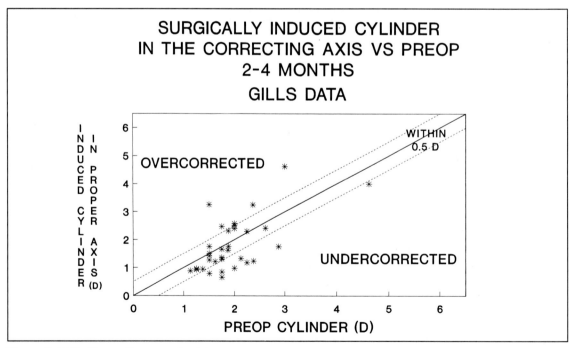

Figure 3-13B. Two to four month visit.

Figure 3-13. The component of surgically induced cylinder in the correcting, or proper, axis versus the preoperative cylinder. The correcting axis is defined as 90° away from the preoperative steep cylinder axis. Points above the equivalency line are overcorrected, and points below the line are undercorrected. Points within the dashed lines are within 0.5 D of a spherical correction.

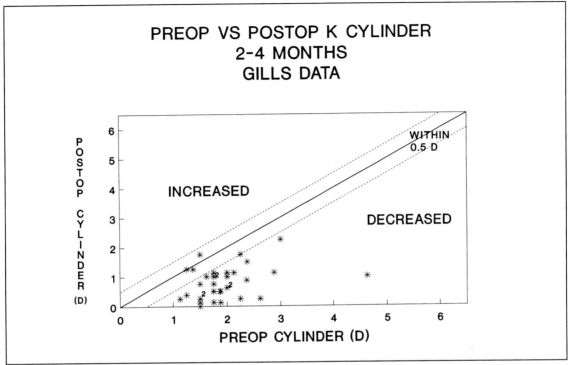

Figure 3-14. Preoperative versus postoperative keratometric cylinder level without regard to axis at the 2-4 month visit. Points above the equivalency line have more cylinder postoperatively and points below have less. Points within the dashed lines are within 0.5 D of preoperative level.

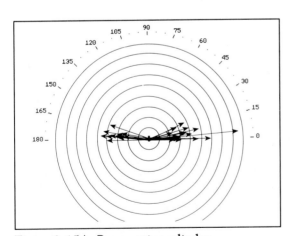

Figure 3-15A. Preoperative cylinder.

Figure 3-15B. Postoperative cylinder.

Figure 3-15. Vector representation of the Gills series. The length of each arrow represents the magnitude of keratometric cylinder and the direction as indicated by the dial represents the steep cylinder axis for each case. Each concentric circle represents 0.5 D.

Topographic Evaluation of Sutureless Cataract Incision at Steep Axis with an Adjacent Arcuate CRI

We at first believed that a single corneal relaxing incision could not be physiologically correct. However, with the use of corneal topography we can see that a single cut will not only flatten at the incision, but also flatten 180° away and steepen in the meridian 90° away. Figure 3-16 demonstrates this effect. The case received a temporal clear-corneal incision with an adjacent CRI. The change map (bottom image) demonstrates asymmetric flattening at the incision site, with some flattening 180° away and steepening 90° away. The postoperative image (top right) shows the astigmatic pattern effectively broken up, and keratometry indicated sphericity.

Interestingly, the patient has both excellent distance and near acuity, an unusual result in a pseudophakic eye. The patient has 20/30 uncorrected acuity, 20/20 corrected acuity, and can see J2 at 14″. Many of the patients receiving a large correction of cylinder seem to have an increased depth of focus. It is possible that steep regions on the cornea postoperatively contribute to a bifocal effect. The topography for this patient indicates isolated steep regions that do not contribute to astigmatism, but may account for a bifocal effect.

Figures 3-17A and 3-17B show the topography of the right and left eyes of a cataract/CRI case. The right eye (Figure 3-17A) received a clear-corneal incision at the steep axis with an

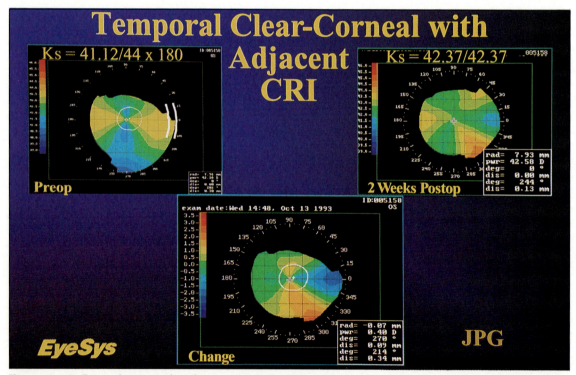

Figure 3-16. Corneal topography of a case receiving a temporal clear-corneal incision with an adjacent CRI. Upper left shows preoperative corneal appearance, upper right shows two week postoperative appearance, and bottom shows surgically induced corneal changes. Note the steep and flat regions on the postoperative image. These concurrent regions may account for this patient's increased depth of focus postoperatively.

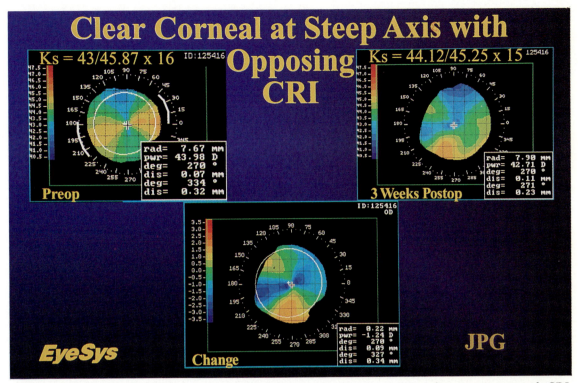

Figure 3-17A. Right eye receiving a clear-corneal incision at the steep axis and an opposing, nasal CRI. Upper left shows preoperative corneal appearance, upper right shows three week postoperative appearance, and bottom shows surgically induced corneal changes.

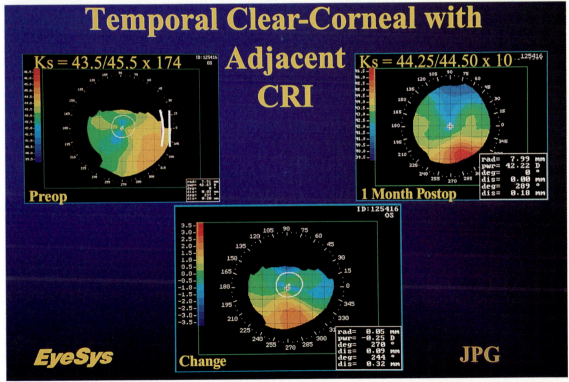

Figure 3-17B. Left eye receiving a temporal clear-corneal incision and adjacent CRI. Upper left shows preoperative corneal appearance, upper right shows one month postoperative appearance, and bottom shows surgically induced corneal changes.

Figure 3-17. Corneal topography of a patient receiving bilateral cataract extraction with CRIs.

opposing nasal CRI to correct 2.87 D of keratometric cylinder. The change map indicates flattening in the meridian of the incisions, with some steepening 90° away. Three weeks postoperatively, the case has a little over 1 D of keratometric cylinder, a correction of over 1.5 D. This patient also has excellent distance and near acuity, seeing 20/25 uncorrected, 20/20 corrected, and J2 at 14″. In this eye there is an inferior steep region on the postoperative image that may account for the increased depth of focus.

The left eye (Figure 3-17B) received a temporal clear-corneal incision with an adjacent CRI to correct asymmetric astigmatism. The change map indicates flattening in the location of the incisions with inferior steepening. Postoperative keratometry indicated only 0.25 D of cylinder. The patient had excellent visual acuity with this eye as well, seeing 20/25 uncorrected and 20/20 corrected. The patient could see J3 at 14″ with this eye. Again, there are steep regions present on the postoperative image, possibly accounting for this effect.

Figure 3-18 shows topography of a case which received a smaller astigmatism correction. A temporal clear-corneal incision and adjacent CRI were performed to correct 1 D of keratometric cylinder. Two months postoperatively, the cylinder was well corrected. Keratometry was 42.75/43.25 x 143, and refraction was plano, with 20/25 uncorrected vision. This patient, however, did not have an increased depth of focus, seeing only J10. As illustrated in the postoperative topography image, the smaller astigmatism correction resulted in a nearly spherical

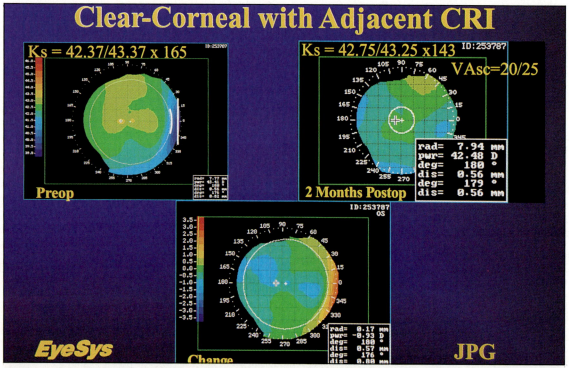

Figure 3-18. Corneal topography of case with 1 D of keratometric cylinder receiving a temporal clear-corneal incision and adjacent CRI. Upper left shows preoperative corneal appearance, upper right shows two month postoperative appearance, and bottom shows surgically induced corneal changes. Note the relatively spherical corneal surface postoperatively. This patient did not experience an increased depth of focus postoperatively.

cornea, without the steep and flat regions which can cause a bifocal effect, seen in the previous cases. It appears that the bifocal effect only occurs in corneas that have at least 2 D of astigmatism preoperatively.

The Thornton Approach

With the Thornton approach, corneal relaxing incisions are not performed at the time of cataract surgery. Instead, the incisions are performed at least three months following the cataract

Table 3-3.
Thornton Nomogram for Arcuate Corneal Relaxing Incisions

One Pair of Arcuate Incisions at the 7-mm OZ

Theoretical Cylinder	Degrees of Arc	Chord Length
0.50 D	20°	1.2 mm
0.75 D	23°	1.3 mm
1.00 D	25°	1.5 mm
1.25 D	28°	1.7 mm
1.50 D	32°	1.9 mm
1.75 D	35°	2.1 mm
2.00 D	38°	2.3 mm
2.25 D	42°	2.5 mm
2.50 D	45°	2.7 mm

Two Pair of Arcuate Incisions

Theoretical Cylinder	Degrees of Arc	Chord Length 6 mm OZ	Chord Length 8 mm OZ
2.00 D	23°	1.2 mm	1.5 mm
2.25 D	27°	1.4 mm	1.8 mm
2.50 D	31°	1.6 mm	2.0 mm
2.75 D	35°	1.8 mm	2.3 mm
3.00 D	39°	2.0 mm	2.6 mm
3.25 D	43°	2.2 mm	2.9 mm
3.50 D	47°	2.4 mm	3.1 mm
3.75 D	48°	2.6 mm	3.3 mm

Three Pair of Arcuate Incisions

Theoretical Cylinder	Degrees of Arc	Chord Length 6 mm OZ	Chord Length 7 mm OZ	Chord Length 8 mm OZ
3.25 D	22°	1.1 mm	1.3 mm	1.5 mm
3.50 D	26°	1.3 mm	1.5 mm	1.8 mm
3.75 D	30°	1.5 mm	1.8 mm	2.1 mm
4.00 D	35°	1.8 mm	2.1 mm	2.4 mm
4.25 D	40°	2.0 mm	2.4 mm	2.7 mm
4.50 D	45°	2.3 mm	2.7 mm	3.1 mm
4.75 D	50°	2.5 mm	3.0 mm	3.4 mm
5.00 D	54°	2.7 mm	3.2 mm	3.6 mm

surgery. In fact, astigmatic keratotomy can be performed years after the cataract surgery, particularly if age and/or cylinder regression from a larger superior incision has resulted in an increase in against-the-rule astigmatism.

Table 3-3 shows the Thornton nomogram. This nomogram uses modifiers—age, sex and intraocular pressure—to the preoperative cylinder to arrive at a "theoretical target cylinder." For every year below age 30 add 0.5% to the cylinder, and for every year above 30 subtract 0.5%. In women below age 40 subtract three years from the actual age. For every mmHg of IOP below 12 add 2% to the cylinder, and for every mmHg above 15 subtract 2%. These modifiers help to improve the predictability of the procedure by accounting for some of the patient-to-patient variability.

Surgical Technique

The Thornton surgical technique for performing arcuate corneal relaxing incisions is described in Chapter 7.

Topographic Evaluation of Arcuate CRIs Performed Post Cataract Surgery

Figure 3-19 shows topography of an 89 year-old woman who had cataract surgery in 1986. She had a 7-mm scleral-tunnel incision closed with two 10-0 nylon X-sutures. She presented in March, 1993 with 3 D of keratometric cylinder. Her refraction was +2.25 -4.50 x 95 with 20/30⁻

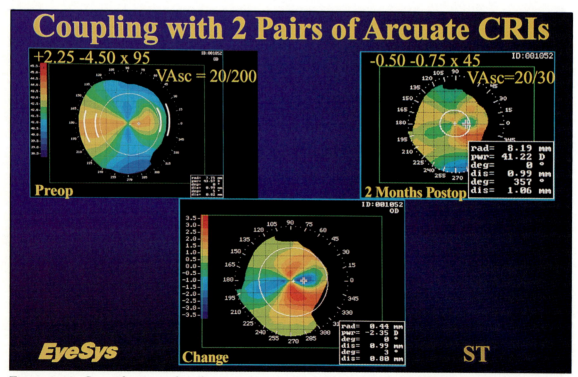

Figure 3-19. Corneal topography of a post-cataract case receiving two pairs of arcuate relaxing incisions. Upper left shows preoperative corneal appearance, upper right shows two month postoperative appearance, and bottom shows surgically induced corneal changes. Note the flattening in the incision meridian combined with steepening 90° away. This effect is called coupling.

best-corrected acuity and 20/200 uncorrected acuity. Two pairs of relaxing incisions were performed at the 6 and 8-mm optical zones. Each incision was 43° of arc. Preoperatively, the topography demonstrated against-the-rule astigmatism. Postoperatively, there appears to be an overcorrection, with some oblique astigmatism. However, the refraction was only -0.50 -0.75 x 45 with 20/30⁻ uncorrected vision and 20/25⁻ best-corrected vision.

Figure 3-20 is the topography of an 89 year-old woman who received cataract surgery in 1982. She had a 7-mm limbal cataract incision closed with three 10-0 nylon X-sutures. She presented in 1992 with moderate against-the-rule astigmatism. Refraction was + 1.00 -4.00 x 90. Due to slight asymmetry in the cylinder power noted on the preoperative topography, two 35° arcuate relaxing incisions were placed nasally and one temporally.

The resulting postoperative refraction at three months was -0.25 -0.75 x 155. The central pupillary area within the white circle in the postoperative image on the right in Figure 3-20 demonstrates a marked reduction in astigmatism. The change graph on the bottom demonstrates more effect nasally where the two incisions were placed.

The 77 year-old male shown in Figure 3-21 had cataract surgery in 1991. He received a 6.5-mm scleral-tunnel incision closed with a single horizontal mattress suture. He presented in 1993 with 3.75 D of refractive cylinder. An undercorrection was planned to match the refraction in the fellow eye. Two relaxing incisions were performed at the 7-mm optical zone. The nasal incision was 40° of arc while the temporal incision was slightly longer, 50° of arc, because the

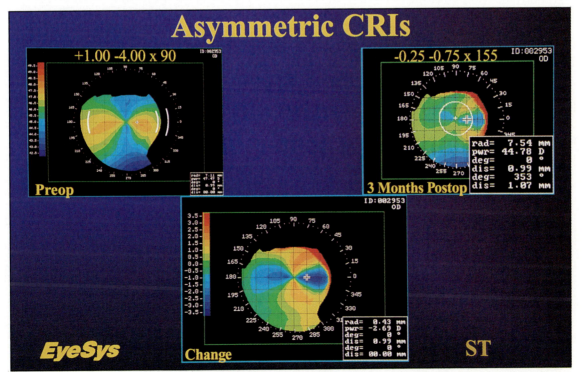

Figure 3-20. Corneal topography of a post-cataract case receiving two relaxing incisions nasally and one temporally. Upper left shows preoperative corneal appearance, upper right shows three month postoperative appearance, and bottom shows surgically induced corneal changes. Note the greater flattening nasally in the change image.

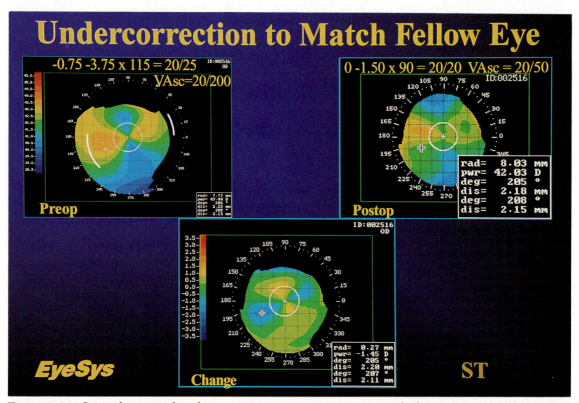

Figure 3-21. Corneal topography of a post-cataract case receiving a pair of relaxing incisions. The surgical plan called for an undercorrection. Upper left shows preoperative corneal appearance, upper right shows postoperative appearance, and bottom shows surgically induced corneal changes.

astigmatism was steeper temporally as shown by topography. Postoperatively the patient had 1.5 D of residual refractive cylinder. Uncorrected visual acuity improved from 20/200 preoperatively to 20/50 postoperatively, with 20/20 best-corrected visual acuity.

Summary

The question of what to do about pre-existing and surgically induced cylinder has become one of *when* to do the correction. The answer by the progressive ophthalmologist is more frequently becoming, "at the time of cataract surgery."

For correcting moderate to large amounts of astigmatism, corneal relaxing incisions appear to be safe and effective, and reasonably predictable. Many surgeons agree that against-the-rule cylinder should be aggressively corrected, while with-the-rule cylinder should be approached conservatively to avoid residual against-the-rule cylinder.

4

Excimer Laser Photoastigmatic Keratectomy

COLMAN R. KRAFF, MD
ALAN V. SPIGELMAN, MD
DON JOHNSON, MD
MANUS C. KRAFF, MD

Introduction

Over the past few years clinical trials have been ongoing in the United States. and around the world evaluating the efficacy of the 193-nm excimer laser to reshape the cornea for the correction of myopia in humans. Results from U.S. Phase III FDA trials as well as independent international clinical trials have demonstrated predictable, reproducible results.[1-4]

Myopic corrections with the Visx Twenty-Twenty® excimer laser (Visx Inc., Sunnyvale, CA) are achieved by passing the laser beam through a computer-controlled iris diaphragm. With each pulse of the laser approximately 0.3 microns of stromal tissue is removed. The effect of the photorefractive keratectomy (PRK) treatment is a cornea that has been ablated to a greater degree in the center than the periphery. United States FDA clinical trials allow spherical myopia treatment if the patient has up to 1.0 D of astigmatism.[3] Although a significant number of patients qualify for PRK treatment, the number of patients with either compound myopic astigmatism of greater than 1.0 D of cylinder, induced post-extracapsular cataract extraction astigmatism, and disabling post-keratoplasty astigmatism is great. In the past, conventional surgical approaches for the correction of astigmatism involved incisional procedures.[5-8] Recently, clinical trials have been underway in the U.S. that are evaluating the efficacy of toric ablations for compound myopic astigmatism as well as postoperative induced astigmatism utilizing the 193-nm excimer laser. This chapter will discuss the software and hardware, patient selection and technique, as well as postoperative results for correcting astigmatism with photoastigmatic refractive keratectomy (PARK) utilizing the Visx Twenty-Twenty excimer laser.

Theory

In 1983 Trokel et al. demonstrated that smooth ablations of the cornea could be produced with the 193-nm excimer laser.[9] Using a pulsed, deep ultraviolet 193-nm ArF excimer laser, corneal ablations were produced with high precision and little damage to the surrounding adjacent corneal stroma. Because of the high energy absorption by the proteins and water components of the stromal tissue, the superficial penetration depth (1-4 microns) allows for production of very smooth ablated surfaces, preserving the optical qualities of the cornea that are essential for good visual acuity.[10] Numerous prospective clinical trials have demonstrated the efficacy of this technology for the treatment of myopia with a high level of predictability.[3,4,11,12] Other applications of the laser are therapeutic in nature and include corneal scarring, dystrophies, and recurrent erosions of the cornea.

The use of the excimer laser for the treatment of myopia relies on either expanding or constricting the iris diaphragm to produce radially symmetric spherical ablations. The center of the cornea is flattened by the delivery of more energy to the center of the treatment zone than the periphery (Figure 4-1), thus removing more stromal tissue from the center of the cornea than the periphery.

Treatment of corneal astigmatism requires selective flattening of the steeper meridian and, depending on the refractive error, concomitant treatment of myopia. Currently, in the U.S., there are two excimer laser systems (Visx Twenty-Twenty and Summit Excimed 2000) that are actively being tested in FDA-approved clinical trials. Both systems require software and hardware adjustments in order to produce cylindrical and spherocylindrical ablations.

The Summit excimer laser has attempted to treat astigmatism with the use of a toric erodible mask. The theory behind the erodible mask is to control the corneal shape in a transfer process. The theoretical advantages of this type of system to treat toric corneal surfaces is the ability to transfer any shape onto the corneal surface, the ability to produce a smoother ablation, potentially easier eye fixation, and treatment in a controlled, humidified environment. The mask is made up of a polymethylmethacrylate material mounted to a transparent quartz plate. The plate is placed onto a plastic shell that is fixated to the limbus via suction.[13] European trials are currently underway, as well as early phase FDA trials in the U.S.

The Visx excimer laser utilizes a different approach to correct astigmatism. The Visx Twenty-Twenty system incorporates modifications of their original hardware and software in order to broaden the range of treatment to include astigmatism and compound myopic astigmatism.

The new hardware consists of a dual aperture system, an iris diaphragm that is capable of expanding or constricting (circular aperture), and a pair of parallel adjustable blades (rectangular aperture) that can rotate 360° (Figure 4-2). The large diameter excimer laser beam is passed through this dual system. The blade separation, like the aperture size, is controlled by the computer

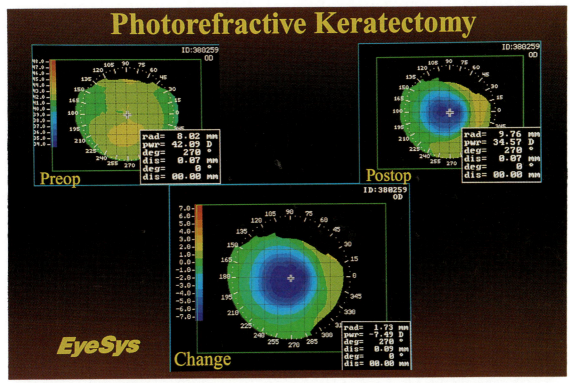

Figure 4-1. Computerized videokeratography of a postoperative photorefractive keratectomy.

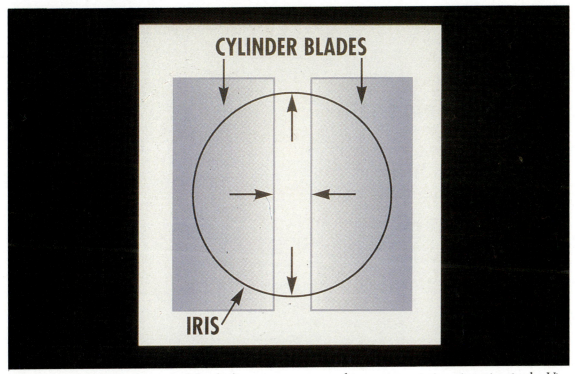

Figure 4-2. Schematic diagram of the dual aperture system used to correct myopic astigmatism in the Visx Twenty-Twenty excimer laser.

software. The slit variability is used to control the amount of ablation in a similar manner to the expanding diaphragm for PRK. The blades are rotated so the long axis (mechanical axis) of the blades are perpendicular to the steep meridian of the cornea (Figure 4-3). No refractive change is intended along the mechanical axis. The computer software controls the rotation of the slits so the mechanical axis is rotated to the same meridian of astigmatism of the patient when expressed in minus cylinder form. For example, if a patient has a refractive error of plano -2.00 x 180, the mechanical axis (long axis) of the blades are rotated to the 180° meridian. The intended flattening, therefore, is to occur along the 90° (steep) meridian.

Using this dual aperture system, blades, and diaphragm, there are two methods by which the Visx excimer laser software is capable of correcting astigmatism alone, as well as compound myopic astigmatism. The first utilizes the two apertures in a sequential manner, the "sequential program." The parallel slits, by changing with each pulse of the laser, produce a rectangular pattern on the cornea (Figure 4-4). The ends of the ablated cylinder are then smoothed with the circular aperture to produce a gradual "transition" zone. This transition is intended to prevent irregular epithelial and stromal healing that could decrease the effective flattening by filling in the ablated area. Any residual myopia can then be treated in a radially symmetric manner using an expanding circular diaphragm. Therefore the "sequential program" is derived, treating astigmatism, then sphere, in sequence.[14]

The second method that the Visx system uses for producing toric ablations produces an elliptical area on the corneal surface, thus the term "elliptical program." In an elliptical ablation

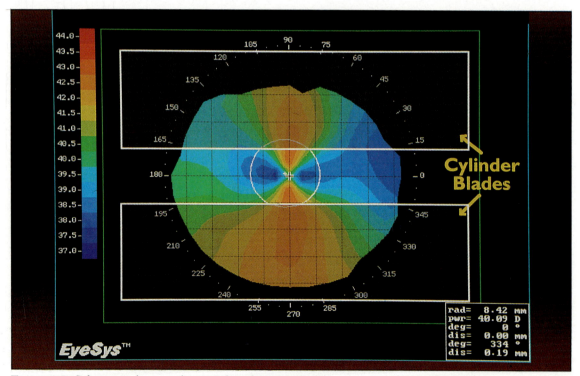

Figure 4-3. Schematic diagram showing the relationship of the mechanical axis of the blades in relationship to the steepest corneal meridian.

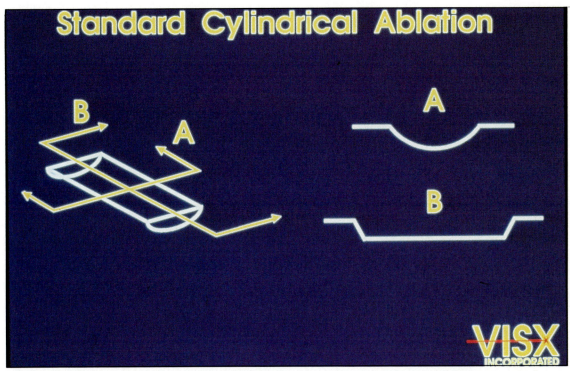

Figure 4-4. Diagram of the rectangular pattern produced on the cornea when treating astigmatism alone.

the astigmatism and sphere are treated simultaneously. The advantage of an elliptical ablation over a sequential ablation is smoother ablation with no transition zones.[15] As can be seen in Figure 4-5, an ellipse has a major and minor axis. The relative sizes of the major and minor axis will depend on the ratio of the cylindrical to spherical correction. The major axis is the axis of the cylinder. To be clinically effective, an elliptical ablation must have a minor axis large enough in diameter so as not to produce any glare when the pupil dilates in dim illumination. The diameter of the minor axis will vary depending on the amount of astigmatism. The greater the degree of astigmatism the smaller the diameter of the minor axis. At the time of this study the largest diameter of treatment with the Visx excimer laser was 6.0 mm. Therefore, if the major axis of the ellipse is held constant at 6.0 mm then the smallest diameter of the minor axis is a minimum of 4.5 mm (Figure 4-6). As a result of this minimum requirement, elliptical ablations have upper limits with respect to the dioptric amount of cylinder being treated. The amount of cylinder can be no greater than the sphere when expressed in minus cylinder form. In patients with cylinder greater than the power of the sphere (minus cylinder form), it is best to treat using the sequential program, thereby minimizing the potential problem of glare in dim illumination.[15] The amount of stroma removed per diopter of myopia and astigmatism are determined by the equations of Munnerlyn which are intrinsic to the astigmatic software.[15,16]

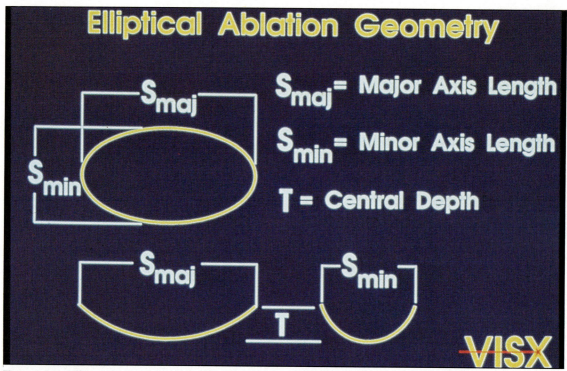

Figure 4-5. Elliptical pattern produced by an elliptical ablation. Note the major and minor axis.

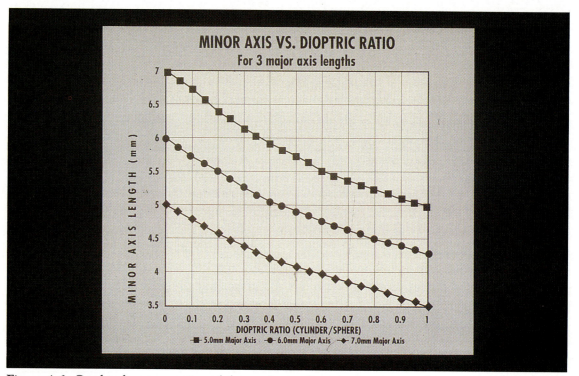

Figure 4-6. Graphical representation of the maximum dioptric correction with an elliptical ablation at varying changes in the diameter of the minor axis.

Materials and Methods

Astigmatism Protocols

Visx, in cooperation with the Food and Drug Administration, is currently investigating photoastigmatic refractive keratectomy (PARK). Phase I and Phase II testing have now been completed. Phase I included ten partially sighted eyes. During Phase IIa testing, twenty-five patients were treated in the U.S. The treatments were performed at five different sites with each site performing five treatments. The patients treated in Phase IIa had between 0.75 and 4 D of astigmatism and up to 6 D of myopia. Phase II patients were followed for six months, after which time the second eye could be treated. Upon completion of follow-up for one year, Phase IIb testing was started which included an additional seventy-five patients at the same sites. Upon completion of Phase IIb, Phase III testing will begin.

In addition to the above FDA Phase II protocol for photoastigmatic refractive keratectomy, patients with unusual refractive abnormalities were treated under a subgroup protocol of phototherapeutic keratectomy (PTK group 2) Phase III testing. PTK group 2 includes patients that had residual postoperative myopia and or astigmatism after penetrating keratoplasty, cataract surgery, or radial keratotomy. Also, patients that have clinically significant anisometropia may be included in this category. The preoperative evaluation, treatment technique, and postoperative follow-up is basically identical to those patients that are treated under the PARK Phase II trial. Results of some of these patients will be reported separately below.

Preoperative Evaluation

All patients in the study went through a series of rigorous preoperative tests. The following tests were carried out for each patient:
- Uncorrected visual acuity
- Manifest and cycloplegic refraction
- Slit lamp examination
- Dilated fundus examination
- Intraocular pressure
- Corneal topography and keratometry
- Corneal pachymetry
- Glare testing
- Contrast sensitivity
- Visual fields
- Specular microscopy

In addition to the tests listed above, a determination was made that the refraction had to be stable over a period of one to two years. Any contact lens wearer had to discontinue lens wear for two weeks prior to evaluation. Throughout each of these evaluations, patients who had any abnormal findings were eliminated from the study. Corneal topography was used to screen for "forme fruste keratoconus" and those patients exhibiting it were eliminated from the study. The criteria used to determine forme fruste keratoconus were those noted by Rabinowitz and McDonnell.[17]

Surgical Technique

The laser was readied by entering the desired refractive change along with the average keratometry into the menu-driven software. The sequential or elliptical programs were used depending on the amount of myopia and astigmatism. A test block of polymethylmethacrylate was ablated and the resulting refractive change verified with a lensometer. Adjustments were made in the laser energy output until the desired refractive change was achieved in the test plastic.

The patients were instructed in detail as to what they would experience during the procedure. Patients were premedicated with up to 20 mg of oral valium depending on body size and sex. During Phase II testing, an axial alignment tool was installed at some of the centers. Patients that were going to participate in a subjective alignment technique were shown a video preoperatively that enabled them to subjectively determine their preoperative axis at the time of treatment. The patients were positioned under the laser and their heads were immobilized with a suction pillow. Those that were participating in the subjective alignment would adjust the astigmatic laser beam with their axis of astigmatism.

After the eye was prepped with betadine solution, a 7-mm optical zone marker was used to center around the visual axis while the patient was fixating on the fixation light in the operating microscope. A 6-mm Merocel sponge which had been soaked in 1/2% topical tetracaine was then placed on the corneal epithelium for one minute. The epithelium was then scraped with a blunt spatula. The patient was instructed to re-focus on the fixation light and asked to continue to fixate throughout the procedure. The surgeon then aimed the center of the laser reticule at the center of the patient's pupil and the laser focused on the corneal surface. The laser was activated with the foot pedal.

Ablation time took between 30 to 60 seconds. The laser treatment could be interrupted at any time by disengaging the foot pedal if any gross loss of fixation occurred. The computer software then allowed completion of the procedure after the patient's eye was realigned. Fortunately, this event rarely occurred.

Postoperative Care

Following surgery, the patients were either patched with TobraDex ointment or placed in a bandage contact lens and started on TobraDex drops four times a day in conjunction with a non-steroidal anti-inflammatory drop, also four times a day. Patients were watched on a daily basis until re-epithelialization occurred. Although the topical non-steroidal drops are very effective in decreasing the postoperative pain, excessive use may impair re-epithelialization. Once re-epithelialization had occurred, typically in 48 to 96 hours, the patients were switched to a regimen

of FML four times a day. The topical drops were continued in a tapering fashion as follows:
- 4 times a day for one month
- 3 times a day for one month
- 2 times a day for one month
- 1 time a day for one month
- every other day for one month

At the conclusion of this five month course, all eye drops were discontinued. In addition to routine refraction, slit lamp and dilated fundus examinations, corneal topography was routinely performed on all patients at one, three and six months postoperatively.

Clinical Results

This section will summarize the clinical results of patients treated at several sites throughout North America. Some of the data are from the 70 consecutive patients for whom at least six month follow-up was completed in Phase II of the FDA clinical trial.

Re-epithelialization occurred between two and six days postoperatively. The postoperative reaction to pain was variable. It was clear that patients who wore a bandage contact lens and used topical non-steroidal anti-inflammatory agents were more comfortable in the immediate postoperative period. In some of the patients that were treated in their first eye with a patch and their second eye with the combination of contact lens and topical non-steroidal agent, there was a clear improvement in postoperative pain.

Table 4-1 summarizes the six month results on the first consecutive seventy patients treated in Phase II of the FDA clinical trial. Table 4-2 summarizes the twelve patients that are at least one year postoperative. The average preoperative sphere was -4.96 D with the average preoperative cylinder -1.52 D. The average postoperative sphere at six months was 0.14 D with an average postoperative cylinder of 0.54 D (Table 4-1). Table 4-2 shows the average preoperative and postoperative sphere and cylinder at twelve months for twelve patients. The uncorrected visual acuity showed that 71% of the patients were 20/40 or better at six months. At one year 83% were 20/40 or better (Table 4-3). The best-corrected visual acuity at six months and one year are demonstrated in Table 4-4. At one year, the postoperative spherical equivalent ranged from +1.50 D to -1.50 D (Figure 4-7). At one year the residual cylinder varied from 0 to 2.00 D (Figure 4-8). At one year two patients lost one line of best-corrected vision and three patients gained one line of best-corrected vision (Figure 4-9). According to the PERK four-year paper, anything less than two lines of best-corrected visual acuity change is within measurement error.[18]

Table 4-5 illustrates the results of 26 consecutive patients that were treated according to PTK group 2 protocol that have three to six month postoperative data. The range of myopia and astigmatism vary to a greater degree than the patients treated under PARK Phase II study because these patients were qualified secondary to their clinically significant anisometropia, residual myopia after a PKP, or residual myopia and astigmatism after radial keratotomy.

A third series of data is presented here from Don Johnson, MD, of New Westminster, BC. At the time of this writing, these data represent the largest series of consecutive astigmatic

Table 4-1.
Results at Six Months Following Photoastigmatic Refractive Keratectomy

Average Preoperative Sphere	-4.96 D
Average Preoperative Cylinder	-1.52 D
Average Postoperative Sphere	-0.14 D
Average Postoperative Cylinder	-0.54 D
N = 70	

Table 4-1. Summary of six month data of 70 consecutive patients.

Table 4-2.
Results at 1 Year Following Photoastigmatic Refractive Keratectomy

Average Preoperative Sphere	-3.85 D
Average Preoperative Cylinder	-1.19 D
Average Postoperative Sphere	-0.05 D
Average Postoperative Cylinder	-0.59 D
N = 12	

Table 4-2. Spigelman, et al. data: one year clinical results.

Table 4-3.
Uncorrected Visual Acuity Following Photoastigmatic Refractive Keratectomy

	6 Months	1 Year
20/20 +	25%	33%
20/40 +	71%	83%
20/200 or worse	5%	0%
Number of Patients	70	12

Table 4-3. Uncorrected visual acuity data (Spigelman, et al.).

Table 4-4.
Best-Corrected Visual Acuity Following Photoastigmatic Refractive Keratectomy

	6 Months	1 Year
20/20 +	47%	83%
20/40 +	95%	100%
20/200 or worse	0%	0%
Number of Patients	70	12

Table 4-4. Best corrected visual acuity data (Spigelman, et al.).

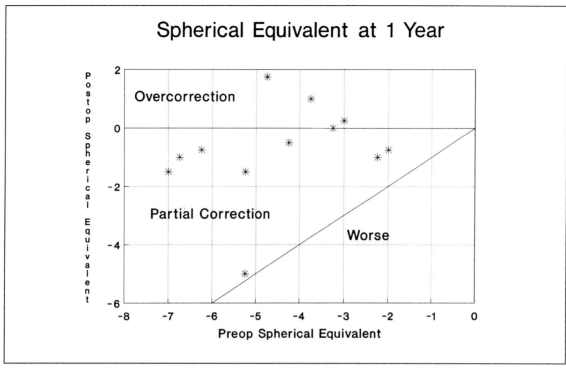

Figure 4-7. Range of spherical equivalent at one year in the FDA clinical trial.

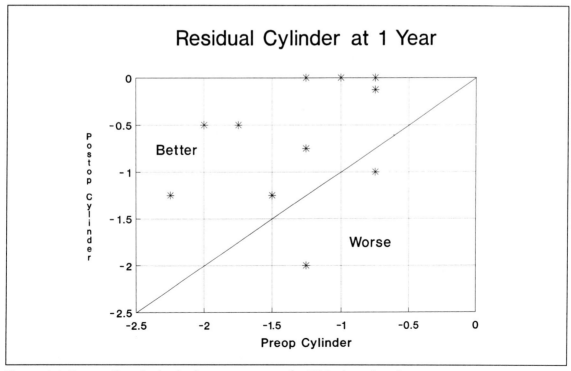

Figure 4-8. Range of residual cylinder at one year in the FDA clinical trial.

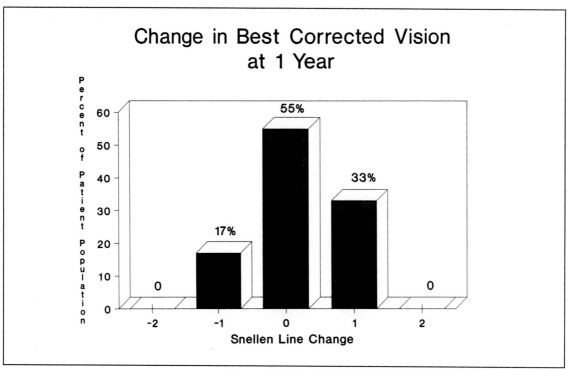

Figure 4-9. Change in best-corrected visual acuity in the FDA clinical trial.

patients treated in the world using the Visx Twenty-Twenty excimer laser. The protocol for treatment was virtually identical to that used in the U.S. clinical trials.

The data are divided into two groups: those treated with elliptical ablations, and those treated with sequential ablations. Figures 4-10A and 4-10B demonstrate the change in mean spherical equivalent over time for both treatment groups. The average change in cylinder is represented in Figure 4-11, and the uncorrected visual acuity is represented in Figures 4-12A and 4-12B. The data demonstrate that patients treated using a sequential treatment program had a higher rate of 20/40 uncorrected vision. They also had almost 1 D more preoperative myopia, which might explain some of the difference.

Topography

Corneal topography has become an essential tool in evaluating patients preoperatively and postoperatively in all keratorefractive procedures, especially in patients undergoing a PARK procedure. Figures 4-13 through 4-16 represent a variety of patients that have undergone either a sequential or elliptical procedure.

The clinical results are highlighted by computerized videokeratography. The images in the upper left corner demonstrate the preoperative corneal evaluation. The images on the left reflect the postoperative image after either an elliptical or sequential program. The lower image is the digital subtraction graph from the preoperative and postoperative images. All patients in these

Table 4-5.
Photoastigmatic Refractive Keratectomy—Kraff Series

Elliptical Patient Data

Preop Refraction	Postop Refraction	Preop UCVA	Postop UCVA	Preop BCVA	Postop BCVA	Months Postop
-3.00 +1.25 x 180	-0.25 +0.25 x 180	20/125	20/25	20/20	20/25	6
-7.50 +1.50 x 90	-0.50 +0.50 x 45	CF	20/30	20/20	20/15	6
-5.25 +2.25 x 85	plano	CF	20/20	20/15	20/20	6
-7.50 +2.50 x 65	-0.25 sphere	CF	20/40	20/20	20/40	6
-3.00 +1.25 x 180	-0.75 sphere	20/100	20/50	20/20	20/25	3
-16.50 +2.50 x 125	plano	CF	20/80	20/100	20/60	3
-4.25 +1.50 x 135	-0.25 +0.25 x 105	20/200	20/20		20/20	3
-2.00 +1.50 x 105	-0.25 +0.25 x 80	20/80	20/20	20/20	20/20	6
-4.50 +2.25 x 90	plano +1.00 x 75	20/100	20/30	20/20	20/20	3
-8.00 +1.25 x 95	-0.25 sphere	CF	20/60	20/20	20/30	3
-4.50 +2.00 x 70	-0.25 +0.25 x 80	CF	20/20	20/20	20/20	6
-7.25 +1.50 x 90	plano 0.50 x 45	CF	20/30	20/20	20/20	3
-8.00 +1.50 x 90	plano +1.00 x 120	CF	20/30	20/20	20/20	3
-4.25 +1.25 x 100	-0.75 +1.00 x 90	20/200	20/40	20/20	20/20	3
-5.25 +2.25 x 85	-0.25 sphere	CF	20/25	20/30	20/20	3
-3.00 +1.50 x 90	1.00 +2.00 x 85		20/100	20/60	20/40	3
-6.75 +1.75 x 110	0.25 sphere	CF	20/50	20/40	20/30	3
-6.00 + 1.00 x 90	-2.25 +0.75 x 65	CF	20/100	20/20	20/25	4
-7.25 +1.50 x 95	plano	CF	20/20	20/20	20/20	6
-4.50 +2.50 x 80	-0.50 +0.25 x 125	20/200	20/25	20/20	20/20	6

Sequential Patient Data

Preop Refraction	Postop Refraction	Preop UCVA	Postop UCVA	Preop BCVA	Postop BCVA	Months Postop
-1.25 +4.00 x 90	-2.50 +6.00 x 180	20/63	20/125	20/40	20/50	6
8.50 +6.00 x 90	13.00 +0.75 x 165	CF	CF	20/100	20/20	3
-5.00 +3.50 x 60	-0.75 +1.00 x 70	20/50	20/30	20/30	20/30	3
plano +6.25 x 135	-1.00 +1.25 x 165	20/200	20/100	20/200	20/100	3
-9.00 +6.00 x 90	-1.00 +1.00 x 30	CF	20/40	20/20	20/40	6
-0.75 +1.75 x 94	-0.50 +0.50 x 80	20/70	20/20	20/20	20/20	6

Table 4-5. Kraff data for patients treated under PTK group 2 protocol.

studies were evaluated preoperatively and postoperatively with EyeSys (Houston, TX) computerized videokeratography. Any residual astigmatism is readily identified and can be used to follow postoperative changes.

Topographical Case Studies
Figure 4-13 demonstrates the topography of a 19 year-old female status post penetrating keratoplasty for keratoconus. Past ocular history was significant for congenital nystagmus, strabismus, and foveal hypoplasia. Postkeratoplasty the patient was intolerant to rigid contact

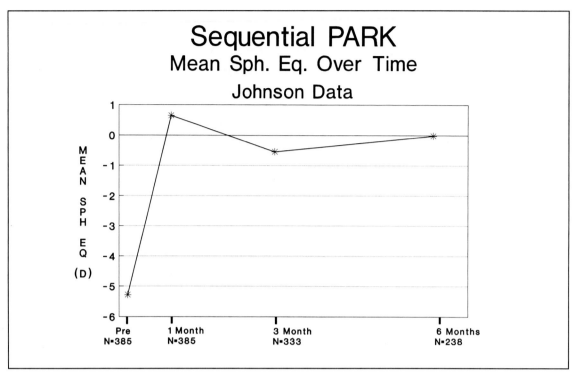

Figure 4-10A. Sequential treatment group.

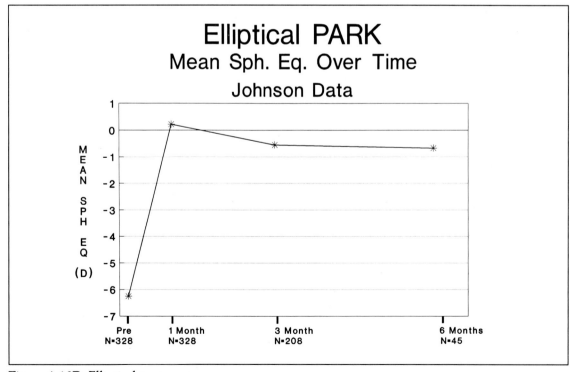

Figure 4-10B. Elliptical treatment group.

Figure 4-10. Mean change in spherical equivalent over time in the Johnson series.

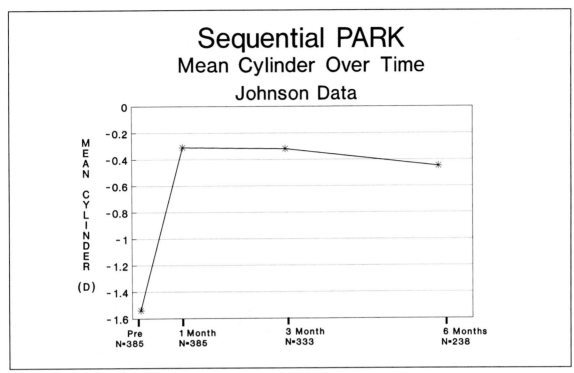

Figure 4-11A. Sequential treatment group.

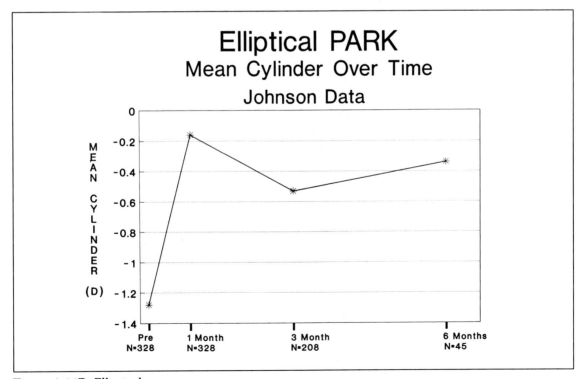

Figure 4-11B. Elliptical treatment group.

Figure 4-11. Mean change in cylinder over time in the Johnson series.

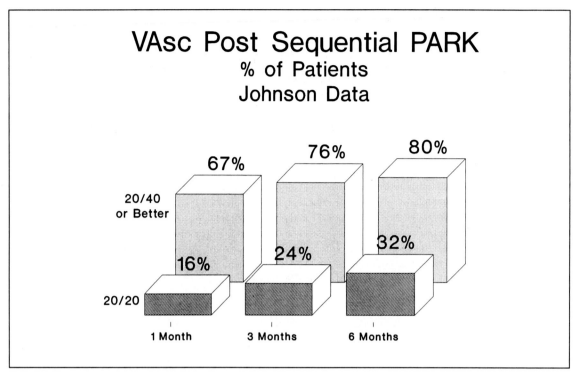

Figure 4-12A. Sequential treatment group.

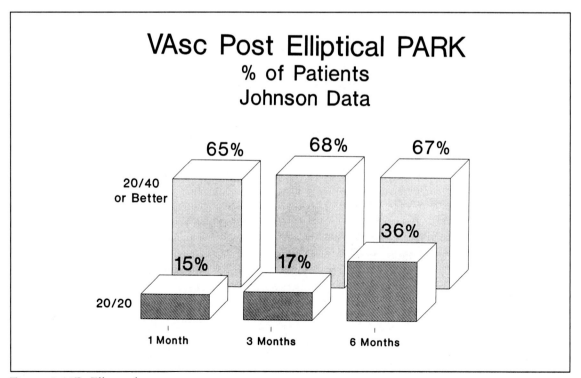

Figure 4-12B. Elliptical treatment group.

Figure 4-12. Percent of patients with uncorrected visual acuity of 20/40 or better in the Johnson series.

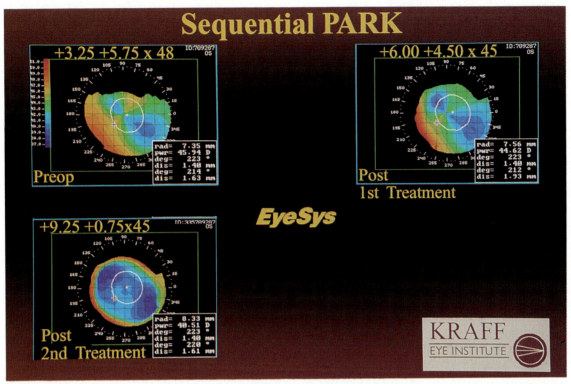

Figure 4-13A. Corneal appearance prior to excimer treatment (upper left), two and a half months following sequential ablation (right), and one month following retreatment with the sequential program (bottom left).

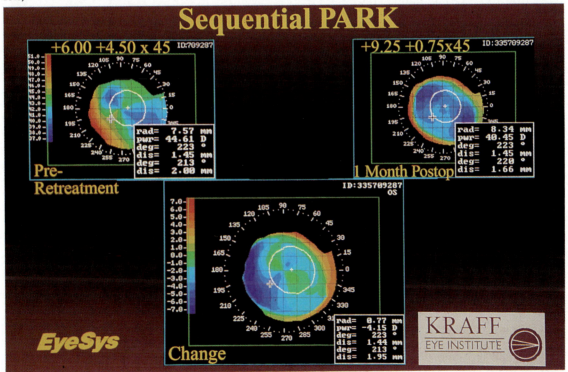

Figure 4-13B. Upper left shows corneal appearance prior to retreatment, upper right shows one month following retreatment with the sequential program, and the bottom image demonstrates the induced corneal change.

Figure 4-13. Corneal topography of a 19 year-old female status post penetrating keratoplasty for keratoconus, with a history of congenital nystagmus, strabismus, and foveal hypoplasia.

lenses and had poor vision with soft toric lenses. Refraction was $+3.25 +5.75$ x 48 with 20/60 best-corrected vision. It was felt that due to the patient's past ocular history her best potential vision was 20/60. She had a strong desire to wear contact lenses.

The patient was treated under the PTK group 2 protocol. The goal was to eliminate as much postkeratoplasty astigmatism as possible. The software setting in the Visx laser for sequential ablation with astigmatism only correction was plano -5.75 x 140, with excimer or transepithelial removal of the epithelium.

Two and a half months postoperatively the refraction was $+6.00 +4.50$ x 45. The possible causes for undercorrection include: alignment error, poor centration, under-estimation of keratometric cylinder secondary to difficulties of refraction from nystagmus, and regression of effect. The patient was subsequently retreated. The retreatment was based on the refraction as well as the topography after the patient had received a retrobulbar block. The software setting was plano 6.00 x 140, with manual epithelial removal. The last available postoperative refraction was $+9.25 +0.75$ x 45, with 20/60 best-corrected vision.

Figure 4-14 shows the topography of a 28 year-old male status post 16-cut radial keratotomy for myopia. The patient was significantly undercorrected at one year postoperatively. Refraction was -4.50 $+2.50$ x 88 with 20/20 best-corrected vision.

The patient was treated under the PTK group 2 protocol for residual myopic astigmatism after radial keratotomy. The software setting for elliptical treatment was -2.44 -2.32 x 180. Postoperatively the refraction was plano $+0.75$ x 180 with $20/20^{+2}$ best-corrected vision. Note that the bottom change graph has greatest flattening in the vertical meridian.

Figure 4-15 demonstrates the topography of a 29 year-old male with myopic astigmatism. Preoperatively, the refraction was -4.00 $+2.00$ x 70 with $20/25^{+2}$ best-corrected vision. The patient was treated with an elliptical program with a setting of -2.67 -1.84 x 160. Postoperatively the refraction was -0.25 $+0.25$ x 80 with 20/20 best-corrected vision. Again, note the vertical pattern of flattening in the change graph, corresponding to the area of steepness postoperatively.

Figure 4-16 shows topography of a 40 year-old male one year status post penetrating corneal laceration, resulting in repair of the laceration followed by a pars plana lensectomy and vitrectomy. The patient was intolerant to aphakic contact lenses with refraction of $+8.50$ $+6.00$ x 90 with 20/100 best-corrected vision. A hard contact lens over the refraction yielded a best-corrected vision of 20/60. The fundus was within normal limits. The remaining remnant of the posterior capsule was 270° around.

The treatment plan was to treat the entire corneal astigmatism with the sequential program, followed by implantation of a posterior chamber intraocular lens at a future date. The software parameters were plano -5.58 x 180 with a treatment zone of 6.0 x 4.5-mm.

Six months following the excimer treatment, the patient's refraction was $+13.00 +1.00$ x 165 with 20/20 best-corrected vision. After implantation of a posterior chamber IOL onto the remaining posterior capsule, the refraction was -0.50 $+2.25$ x 180 with 20/20 best-corrected vision. The topographical change image (bottom) demonstrates the induced flattening following the same pattern where the preoperative topography indicated steepness.

Elliptical PARK

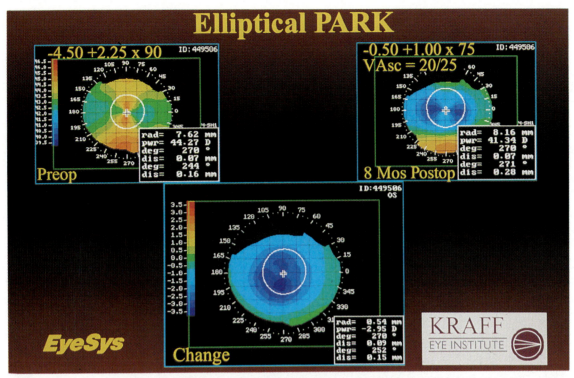

Figure 4-14. Topography of a 28 year-old male status post 16-incision radial keratotomy receiving photoastigmatic refractive keratectomy with an elliptical ablation. Upper left shows pre-ablation, upper right shows post-ablation, bottom shows induced changes.

Elliptical PARK

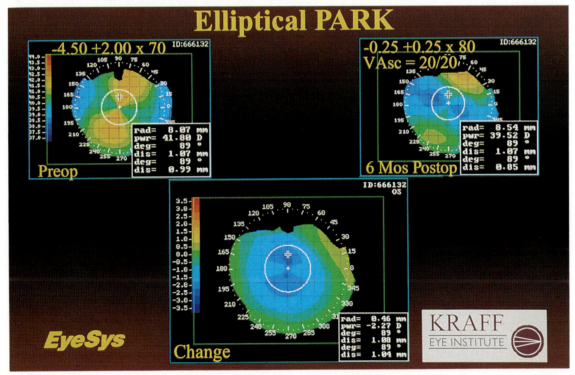

Figure 4-15. Topography of a 29 year-old male receiving photoastigmatic refractive keratectomy with an elliptical ablation for myopic astigmatism. Upper left shows pre-ablation, upper right shows post-ablation, bottom shows induced changes.

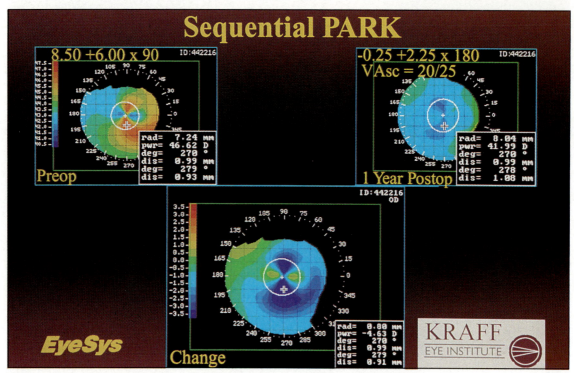

Figure 4-16. Topography of a 40 year-old male status post repair of corneal laceration, pars plana lensectomy, and vitrectomy. Upper left shows pre-ablation, upper right shows post-ablation, bottom shows induced changes.

Discussion

In the past, the surgical correction of astigmatism relied primarily on corneal relaxing incisions of some type. The numerous techniques for either naturally occurring or surgically induced astigmatism suggest that there is not one procedure that is superior than another for all patients. A number of variables such as corneal wound healing, patient age, and technique variability from surgeon to surgeon all probably play a role in the relative lack of predictability.[6-8]

With the development of the excimer laser, the goals were to produce a safe, relatively automated, easily learned, and predictable procedure to correct both myopia and astigmatism. The results from Phase I, II, and III FDA clinical trials suggest that PRK is indeed a predictable, safe procedure for the correction of myopia for -1.0 to -6.0 D with 1 D or less of astigmatism.[1-4] Whether this technology will someday make manual keratorefractive procedures for myopia obsolete is yet to be determined. The photoastigmatic keratectomy trials were designed to further expand the role of the excimer laser to include correcting astigmatism of greater than 1 D. McDonnell et al. were able to show in initial clinical tests, in animals and then humans, that this procedure had potential for the treatment of astigmatism.[17] The preliminary results of this Phase I and II clinical testing in the U.S. suggest that this is indeed a procedure that is efficacious. In order for it to be accepted as the standard, however, it must be better than conventional surgical approaches for correcting astigmatism. At this point the majority of patients treated had a significant reduction in their preoperative cylinder in combination with a reduction in their myopia. All patients had a marked improvement in their uncorrected visual acuity. There are a number of factors which probably contributed to some of the variability of the results in this series. Corneal wound healing can play a role in regression of the flattening effect. If the ablated corneal surface is not uniformly smooth there is a tendency for the stromal keratocytes to produce collagen to fill in the flattened area. Also, the epithelium may heal irregularly and fill in some of the flattened area.[19-21] This healing response can have several negative effects on the final visual result. First, it may reduce the total flattening effect and therefore produce an undercorrection. Second, an irregular healing response can produce an irregular astigmatism, possibly resulting in a decrease in the best-corrected vision with complaints of glare, ghosting of images, and monocular diplopia. Finally, abnormal corneal healing can result in frank corneal scarring from excessive collagen production which usually requires retreatment. Fortunately this complication rarely occurred. Postoperative steroids and/or combinations with non-steroidal anti-inflammatory agents may play a role in some patients in preventing regression.

Visual axis alignment is another factor that can contribute to the visual outcome. A five to ten degree off-axis shift in treatment from the intended axis of astigmatism can result in an undercorrection of 10-20% (Figure 4-17). This misalignment may result from an error in the preoperative refraction, malposition of the patient's head at the time of surgery, centering error on the part of the operating surgeon, or fixation error on the part of the patient.[22] The nomograms intrinsic to the software for correcting the astigmatic component are believed to undercorrect by

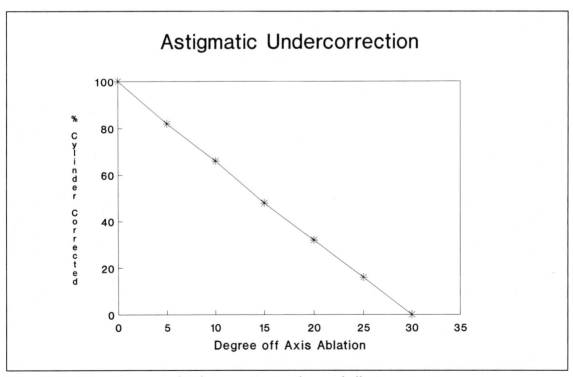

Figure 4-17. Dioptric percent of undercorrections per degree of off-axis treatment.

about 20%.[17,23] Most investigators are now adding a fudge factor of 20% to the astigmatic component in order to compensate for this undercorrection. Eventually software upgrades will automatically compensate for this type of undercorrection in the astigmatic component.

Finally, laser beam quality can contribute to the final refractive result. Poor beam quality either from bad optics (mirror degradation) or calibration errors can produce surface irregularities, central islands (Figure 4-18) (i.e., an area of central steepening with surrounding flat zone) as well as under- and overcorrection. At this time Visx recommends regular maintenance programs. The amount of maintenance will depend on laser usage. In the U.S. where there is significant limitation on the number of procedures performed on each machine, typical maintenance will be about four times per year. Besides regular maintenance checks, prior to each treatment calibration plastics are cut to closely follow beam quality. Any deviation from the predefined intended optical result will trigger a mandatory maintenance call before treatment continues. As experience increases and machines become stressed with increased usage, beam quality maintenance will become more standardized and reliable, eventually leading to improved visual results with less inter-machine variability.

Computerized videokeratography is a relatively new diagnostic tool that allows for accurate preoperative and postoperative evaluation of corneal surface topography of all patients undergoing keratorefractive procedures, and excimer laser surface ablation for myopia and astigmatism in particular. At this time videokeratography is used to screen all patients preoperatively for any abnormal surface topography. With the increased prevalence of computerized videokeratography

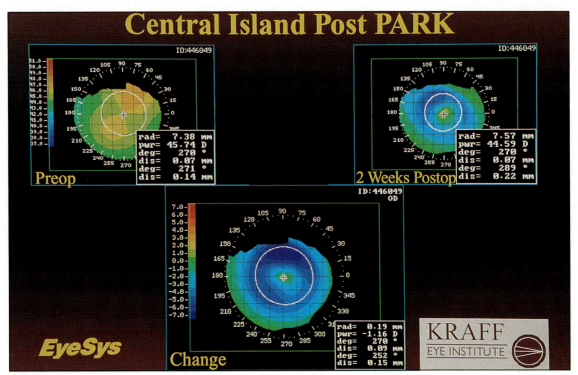

Figure 4-18. Computerized videokeratography of a central corneal island following elliptical PARK.

in patients undergoing keratorefractive surgery, it has become apparent that in some patients, the central cornea will demonstrate more cylinder on topography than is apparent clinically on refraction. Dictum in keratorefractive surgery in the past has been to treat patients according to their cycloplegic refraction. Currently, in Canada and Europe, results of videokeratography are being incorporated into the treatment plan when there is more astigmatism present topographically then is present refractively.[24] Depending on the amount of topographic cylinder, either an elliptical or sequential program is used in order to produce a more spherical postoperative corneal surface. The 20% undercorrection factor as well as an additional amount of cylindrical correction is added in order to achieve the optimal spherical corneal surface. The goal will be to eventually incorporate this type of information directly into the laser software so real-time corneal topography can be incorporated into all photoablative procedures.

The excimer laser for the treatment of astigmatism shows great promise as a potential alternative to conventional methods of astigmatic correction.[25] As surgical experience grows and hardware and software improvements occur, correcting astigmatism with the excimer laser should continue to improve in safety, predictability and patient satisfaction. Eventually, all surgeons will be able to add this new technology to their repertoire for the surgical treatment of astigmatism.

References

1. McDonald MB, Frantz JM, Klyce SD, et al: Central photorefractive keratectomy for myopia: the blind eye study. *Arch Ophthalmol* 108:799-808, 1990.

2. McDonald MB, Liu JC, Bryd TJ, et al: Central photorefractive keratectomy for myopia: partially sighted and normally sighted eyes. *Ophthalmology* 98: 1327-37, 1991.

3. Salz JJ, Maguen E, Nesburn AB, et al: A two year experience with excimer laser photorefractive keratectomy for myopia. *Ophthalmology* 100:873-882, 1993.

4. Seiler T, Wollensak J: Myopic photorefractive keratectomy with the excimer laser: one year follow-up. *Ophthalmology* 98:1156-63, 1991.

5. Swinger CA: Postoperative astigmatism. *Surv Ophthalmol* 31:219-248, 1987.

6. Rowsey JJ: Review: current concepts in astigmatic surgery. *J Refract Surg* 2:85-94, 1986.

7. Laver GW, Lindstrom RL, Hofer LA, Doughman DJ: The surgical management of corneal astigmatism after penetrating keratoplasty. *Opthalmic Surg* 16:165-169, 1985.

8. Villasenor RA, Stimac GR: Clinical results and complications of trapezoidal keratectomy. *J Refract Surg* 4:125-131, 1988.

9. Trokel S, Srinivasan R, Braren B: Excimer laser surgery of the cornea. *Am J Ophthalmol* 96:710-715, 1983.

10. Marshall J, Trokel S, Rothery S, Krueger R: Photoablative reprofiling of the cornea using an excimer laser: photorefractive keratectomy. *Lasers Ophthalmol* 1:21-48, 1986.

11. Tengroth B, Epstein D, Fagerholm P, et al: Excimer laser photorefractive keratectomy for myopia: clinical results of sighted eyes. *Ophthalmol* 100:739-745, 1993.

12. Durrie DS: Clinical results of photorefractive keratectomy for myopia. Presented at the International Society of Refractive Keratoplasty, Anaheim, CA, October 12, 1991.

13. Brancato R, Carones F, Trabucchi G, et al: The erodible mask in photorefractive keratectomy and astigmatism. *Refractive and Corneal Surg* 9(suppl):125-130, 1993.

14. Clapham TN, D'Arcy JD, Bechtel L, et al: Analysis of an adjustable slit design for correcting astigmatism. *SPIE Ophthalmic Technologies* 1423:2-7, 1991.

15. Shimmick J, Bechtel L: Elliptical ablations for the correction of compound myopic astigmatism by photoablation with apertures. *SPIE Ophthalmic Technologies* 1644:32-39, 1992.

16. Rabinowitz YS, McDonnell PJ: Computer assisted corneal topography in keratoconus. *Refract Corneal Surg* 5:400-408, 1989.

17. McDonnell PJ, Hamilton M, Clapham TN, et al: Photorefractive keratectomy for astigmatism: initial clinical results. *Arch Ophthalmol* 109:1370-1373, 1991.

18. Waring GO, Lynn MJ, Fielding B, et al: Results of the Prospective Evaluation of Radial Keratotomy (PERK) study four years after surgery for myopia. *J Am Med Assoc* 263:1083-1091, 1990.

19. Goodman GL, Trokel SL, Stark WJ, et al: Corneal healing following laser refractive keratectomy. *Arch Ophthalmol* 107:1799-1803, 1989.

20. Shieh E, Hamilton M, D'Arcy J, et al: Quantitative analysis of wound healing after cylindrical and spherical excimer laser ablations. *Ophthalmology* 99:1050-1055, 1992.

21. Marshall J, Trokel SL, Rothery S, et al: Long-term healing of the central cornea after photorefractive keratectomy using an excimer laser. *Ophthalmology* 95:1411-1421, 1988.

22. Personal communication. Bill Telfair, Ph.D., Visx Inc., Sunnyvale, CA, October 1993.

23. Personal communication. Don Johnson, M.D., New Westminster, BC, Oct. 22, 1993.

24. Visx Inc. International users meeting, Toronto, Canada, October, 1993.

25. Spigelman AV, Albert WC, Cozean CH, et al: Treatment of myopic astigmatism with the 193 nm excimer laser utilizing aperture elements. Presented at the American Society of Cataract and Refractive Surgery, Seattle, WA, May 12, 1993.

5

Holmium:YAG Laser Thermokeratoplasty for Hyperopic Astigmatism

Daniel S. Durrie, MD
D. James Schumer, MD
Vance M. Thompson, MD

Introduction

With regard to laser use, ophthalmology has remained at the forefront of medical technology since Ruby laser photocoagulation in the 1960s. Today, lasers in ophthalmology range across and beyond the visible electromagnetic spectrum. The excimer laser at 193 nanometers performs ablation of corneal tissue by breaking corneal chemical bonds. Infrared lasers ranging from 1.9 to 2.9 microns create heat through stimulation of water molecules in the tissue. Table 5-1 shows the current list of solid state infrared lasers and their respective wavelengths.

A laser's potential use is determined by its tissue interaction. Solid state infrared lasers have multiple potential uses in ophthalmology. In the field of glaucoma, they are used for both filtering and ciliary destructive procedures. In refractive surgery, infrared lasers are under investigation to treat myopia, hyperopia and astigmatism through thermokeratoplasty.

Throughout this chapter, we will discuss holmium:YAG laser thermokeratoplasty's (HLTK) potential to treat astigmatism. Beginning with historical consideration of thermokeratoplasty and the physiology of corneal tissue interaction to heat, we will address the specific benefits of the holmium:YAG laser. A case study will demonstrate the clinical application of the holmium:YAG laser to treat astigmatism. The challenges for both the surgeon and engineers to further improve and perfect this refractive application will then be discussed.

Thermokeratoplasty History

Thermokeratoplasty was first performed by Lans in 1898. Astigmatism was induced in rabbits with arcuate applications of electrocautery placed parallel to the limbus. He reported a 6 D effect with a 90° arcuate treatment that regressed to 3 D at three months.[1]

In 1984, Fyodorov developed a technique using a nichrome tip probe placed radially in the stroma to 80% depth and heated to 600° C for 0.3 seconds. Termed radial thermokeratoplasty, it corrected hyperopia through stromal collagen shrinkage producing central corneal steepening. Due to the extreme temperatures generated with this procedure, a distinct coagulation profile is seen on histology (Figure 5-1). Centrally, there is necrosis surrounded by an area of collagen relaxation. Collagen shrinkage occurs in the outer most zone. The central corneal steepening is a result of the collagen shrinkage in this outer zone.

Table 5-1.	
Laser Type	**Wavelength**
Cobalt Mg	1.8 to 2.4 microns
Erbium YSGG	2.79 microns
Holmium:YAG	2.1 microns
Thulium:YAG	1.9 microns

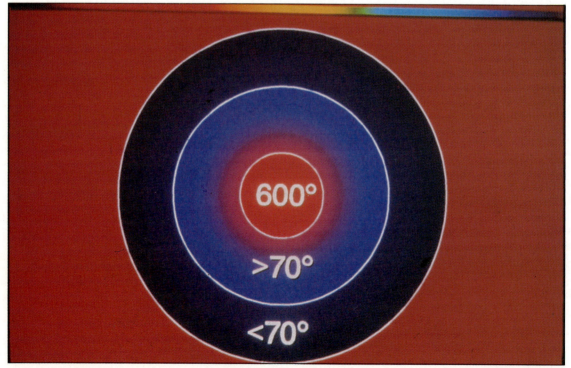

Figure 5-1. Graphical depiction of the temperature zones created with radial thermokeratoplasty. Necrosis occurs in the central zone. Collagen relaxation is produced by the temperature in the intermediate zone, and only in the outer zone does collagen shrinkage occur.

The clinical investigations of radial thermokeratoplasty demonstrated unpredictability and large regressions.[2] An obvious culprit may have been the accompanying collagen necrosis and relaxation that is present in the center of each application. The use of holmium:YAG laser to perform thermokeratoplasty grew out of the need for a uniform thermal delivery system. Theoretically, this system would provide discrete coagulation profiles leading to increased predictability and decreased regression.

Physiology of Collagen Shrinkage

The holmium:YAG laser produces changes in corneal curvature due to its effect on stromal collagen. There is a sequential response of collagen when exposed to increasing temperatures (Figure 5-2). Up to 70° C, collagen denaturation with unraveling of the triple helix occurs. Both the heat labile and heat stable crosslinks remain intact allowing the molecule to recoil from its native elongated state into a contracted state. This phenomenon provides the force of shrinkage. Beyond 70° C, the heat labile crosslinks begin to hydrolyze, allowing relaxation of the collagen molecule from its contracted state, reducing the shrinkage force.[3]

The thermal effect on collagen is both temperature and time dependent. Not only does the temperature need to be precisely controlled, but also the time interval of the thermal application. The holmium:YAG laser produces the appropriate energy (19 mj) at the correct wavelength (2.1 microns) over the precise time interval (1.6 seconds) to provide consistent zones of collagen shrinkage.

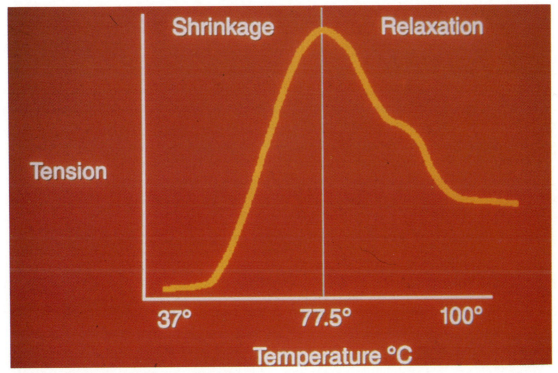

Figure 5-2. Tension graft showing collagen's response to increasing temperatures.

Holmium:YAG Lasers

In search for a laser to cause an appropriate coagulation profile of stromal collagen, a CO_2 laser with a wavelength of 10.6 um provided no refractive change.[4] Due to the cornea absorbing all the energy in the first 60 um, a large enough coagulation profile was not achievable to affect corneal curvature. A Yt-Er-glass laser at a wavelength of 1.54 um did increase corneal curvature significantly but penetration was over 1 mm, raising concern of damage to the endothelium and iris.[5]

Theo Seiler, MD, PhD, was the first to report on holmium:YAG thermokeratoplasty.[6] The holmium:YAG laser with a wavelength of 2.1 um produces corneal steepening without clinical or histological evidence of damage to the endothelium. An additional advantage of the holmium:YAG laser is its ability to titrate the temperature increase. At 19 mj per pulse, 25 pulses, and 15 Hz, a homogeneous coagulation profile without evidence of necrosis is produced.

Summit Technologies of Massachusetts has developed a holmium:YAG laser. The energy of this laser is delivered through a quartz fiber optic handpiece focused by a sapphire tip with a cone angle of 120º (Figure 5-3A and 5-3B). The tip is applied to the corneal surface with the treatment creating a cone of collagen shrinkage measuring 700 um in diameter at the corneal surface and 450 um deep (Figure 5-4).

Sunrise has also developed a holmium:YAG laser. This laser is a non-contact system delivered at a slit lamp (Figure 5-5). Simultaneously, eight applications are delivered producing a half-sphere shaped coagulation profile in the anterior stroma. Figure 5-6 graphically depicts the coagulation profile of both the Summit (Figure 5-6A) and Sunrise (Figure 5-6B) holmium:YAG lasers.

Holmium:YAG Laser Results—Astigmatism

Compound myopic astigmatism is best treated with astigmatic keratotomy. This procedure flattens the steep axis thereby promoting a correction of myopia. In mixed astigmatism or compound hyperopic astigmatism, the goal should be to preserve or enhance corneal steepening. Holmium:YAG thermokeratoplasty, by steepening the flat axis of astigmatism, promotes a hyperopic correction. This effect can be especially important for presbyopic or near presbyopic patients where corneal steepening can lead to good uncorrected near vision.

A total of 30 eyes of 30 patients has been treated in Phase I of Summit Technology's Holmium Astigmatism Laser Thermokeratoplasty Clinical Investigation. With six month follow-up, all patients had a reduction in their refractive astigmatism, 65.5% had an improvement in uncorrected visual acuity, 34.5% had no change, and none had a decrease. No eyes developed keratitis, cataract, corneal decompensation, epithelial defect, ulceration, foreign body sensation, iritis, glare or halos.

Case Presentation

A 52 year-old woman was treated as part of the Summit Technology's Phase I Holmium Astigmatism Laser Thermokeratoplasty Clinical Investigation. She was treated with two pairs of applications at an 8.5-mm optical zone on the flat axis of astigmatism. Her preoperative, two month, four month and six month postoperative refraction, best-corrected visual acuity (BCVA), uncorrected visual acuity (UCVA), and topography are shown in Figures 5-7A and 5-7B.

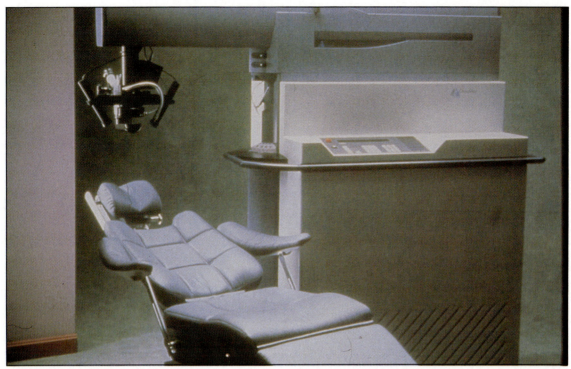

Figure 5-3A. The Summit Technology's Inc. Omnimed laser workstation that contains the holmium:YAG laser.

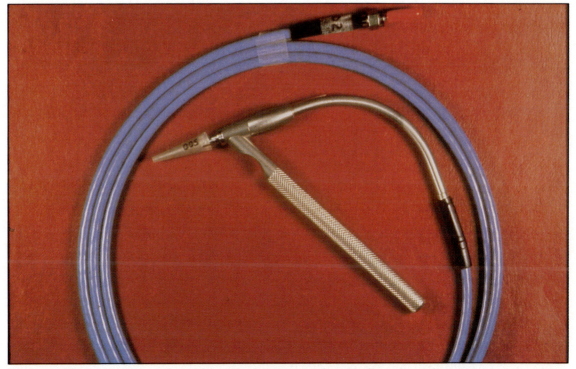

Figure 5-3B. The handpiece that delivers the laser energy through direct corneal contact.

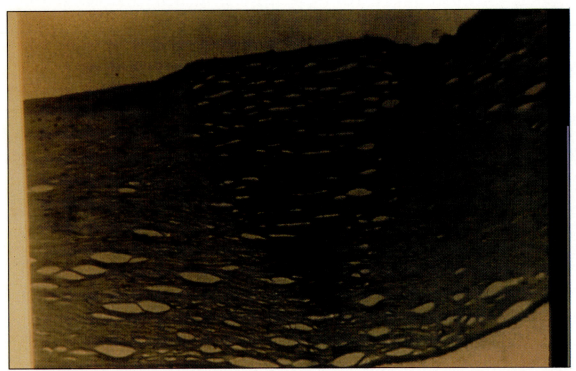

Figure 5-4. Histological preparation showing the corneal stroma coagulation profile of a holmium:YAG laser (used by permission of Theo Seiler, MD).

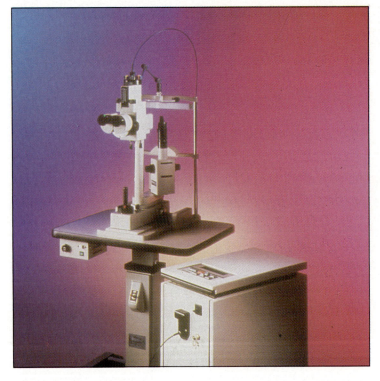

Figure 5-5. Sunrise Technology holmium:YAG laser uses a slit lamp delivery system.

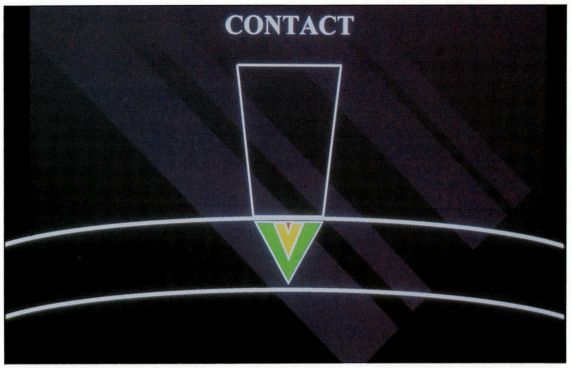

Figure 5-6A. Contact delivery system.

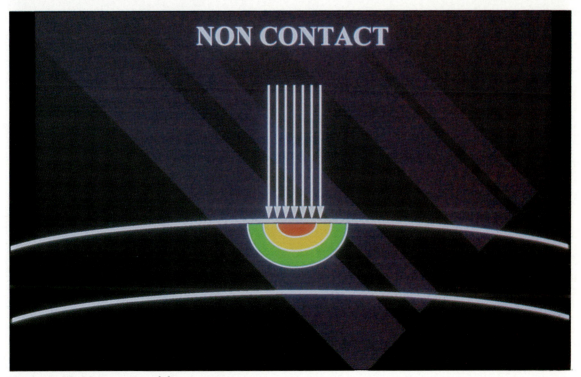

Figure 5-6B. Non-contact delivery system.

Figure 5-6. Graphical depiction of the varying coagulation profiles that result from a contact versus non-contact delivery system.

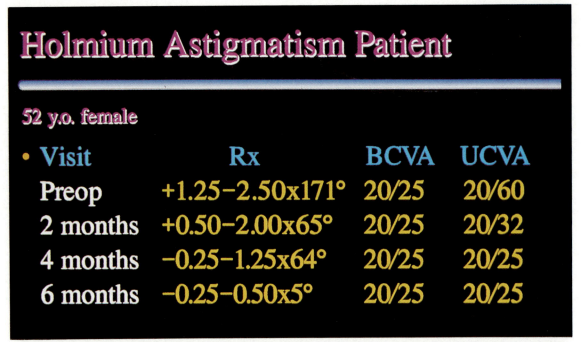

Holmium Astigmatism Patient

52 y.o. female

Visit	Rx	BCVA	UCVA
Preop	+1.25−2.50x171°	20/25	20/60
2 months	+0.50−2.00x65°	20/25	20/32
4 months	−0.25−1.25x64°	20/25	20/25
6 months	−0.25−0.50x5°	20/25	20/25

Figure 5-7A. Preoperative through six months postoperative data on a patient treated in Phase I of Summit Technology's Holmium Astigmatism Laser Thermokeratoplasty Clinical Investigation.

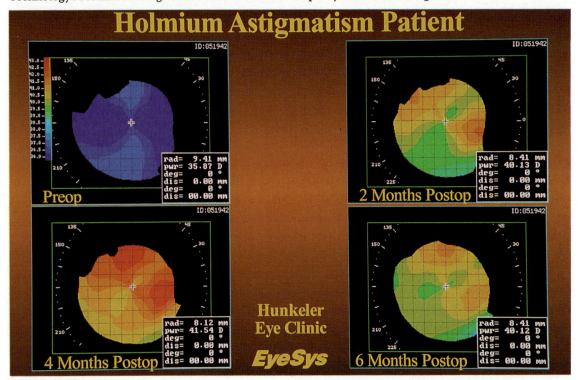

Figure 5-7B. Preoperative, two month, four month, and six month postoperative corneal topography (used by permission of Vance Thompson, MD).

Figure 5-7. Case example.

Challenges for HLTK

As we first determine safety and efficacy for HLTK through the early clinical trials, the studies will expand to treat more patients at more centers. The engineering challenges are to assure the most precise and reproducible coagulation profile. By controlling the temperature over exact time limits through a delivery system that insures a precise profile, damage to adjacent tissues will be prevented while providing maximum effect. Current algorithms and nomograms will expand to include variations for age, sex and numerous other variables that affect outcome. Understanding the biochemical cause for regression will allow for proper treatment and possible prevention through pharmaceutical therapies.

Surgical challenges include identifying the optical axis and maintaining centration throughout the treatment. With Summit's contact technique, the probe tip must be applied perpendicular to the corneal surface with uniform pressure in order to assure consistent coagulation profiles. Decentered or irregular treatment will undoubtedly lead to poor results.

Holmium:YAG laser thermokeratoplasty is a technically simple procedure and the initial results have been encouraging. No refractive surgery procedure can be judged with only six months follow-up. The success of this procedure will rest on larger long-term clinical studies.

References

1. Lans LJ: Experimentelle untersuchungen uber Entstehung von Astigmatismus durch nicht-perforierende Corneawunden. *Arch Ophthalmol* 45:117-152, 1898.

2. Neumann A, Sanders D, Raanan M, et al: Hyperopic thermokeratoplasty: clinical evaluation. *J Cataract Refract Surg* 17:830-838, 1991.

3. Allain J, LeLons M, Cohen-Solal L, et al: Isometric tensions developed during the hydrothermic swelling of rat skin. *Connect Tissue Res* 7:127-133, 1980.

4. Beckman H, Rota A, Barraco R, et al: Limbectomies, keratectomies, and keratotomies performed with rapid-pulsed CO_2 laser. *Am J Ophthalmol* 71:1277-1283, 1971.

5. Kanoda A, Sorokin A: Laser correction of hypermetropic refraction. In Fyodorov S, ed, *Microsurgery of the Eye*. Moscow, Mir Publishers, pp 147-154, 1987.

6. Seiler T, Matallana M, Bende T: Laser thermokeratoplasty by means of a pulsed Holmium:YAG laser for hyperopic correction. *Refract Corn Surg* 6:335-339, 1991.

Section II

Astigmatism Management After Corneal Transplantation

6

Management of Suture-In Astigmatism Following Penetrating Keratoplasty

JOHNNY L. GAYTON, MD
ROGER F. STEINERT, MD

Introduction

Following penetrating keratoplasty, many patients experience severe, visually disabling astigmatism caused by the tension from the sutures. Since these sutures must be left in place for a long time, sometimes as long as five years, it is essential to provide appropriate astigmatic relief so that these patients may have functional vision while the cornea heals. If interrupted sutures are in place, selective suture cutting can relieve the suture-caused tension on the cornea, simultaneously flattening the excessively steep area in the region of the cut suture and steepening the cornea 90° away. As sutures are cut, the remaining sutures can create different patterns of distortion, so the management of the astigmatism becomes an ongoing process until the cornea settles into an acceptable shape that provides reasonably good vision.

If a running suture is necessary for splinting the cornea, tension on the cornea can be relieved by pulling slack suture material from flat areas toward steeper areas. Usually this process is accomplished in many steps over a period of time, allowing the cornea to settle between each suture adjustment, until the tension on the cornea is equalized.

Computer-assisted videokeratography, or corneal topography, is essential for managing suture-in astigmatism. The tension on the cornea often creates asymmetrical or non-orthogonal astigmatism, or isolated steep regions causing severe irregular astigmatism. Keratometry is inadequate for characterizing these types of corneal shape, and Placido images can be difficult to interpret.

Figure 6-1A demonstrates the Placido image of a penetrating keratoplasty case with a tight interrupted suture. It is not obvious from this image where the tight suture is. However, with a color-coded topographical overlay map (Figure 6-1B), the location of the suture that needs removal is easily identified as the marked area of steepening (red region).

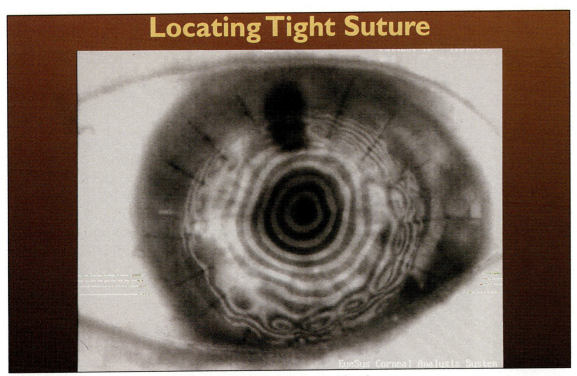

Figure 6-1A. Location of a tight suture is not obvious from a Placido image.

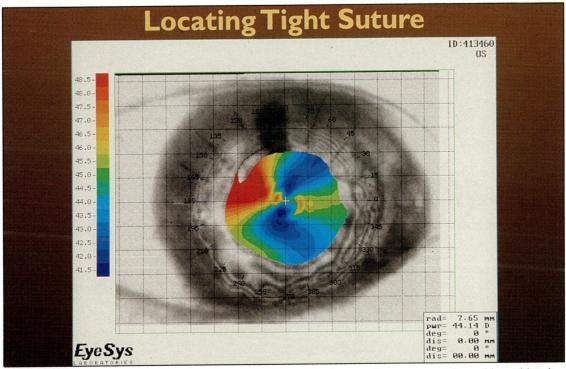

Figure 6-1B. With a color-coded overlay corneal map, marked areas of steepening indicated by red localize the suture(s) that needs removal.

Topographical Case Studies

Case 1: Progressive Reduction in Astigmatism with Improvement in Acuity with Removal of Interrupted Sutures

This 80 year-old gentleman lost his left eye from a traumatic rupture of a previous penetrating keratoplasty. His right eye had penetrating keratoplasty due to progressive pseudophakic decompensation associated with Fuch's dystrophy on February 9, 1993. Because of the history in the fellow eye, suturing was done with 16 interrupted 10-0 Prolene sutures. Prolene is more elastic than nylon and historically has been associated with high degrees of astigmatism.

The patient exhibited an inflammatory reaction to the sutures. Combined with spontaneous loosening of some of his sutures due to the inflammation, and the need to reduce astigmatism to allow useful vision in his only eye, the patient has undergone slow removal of multiple sutures postoperatively, providing a nice illustration of the progressive reduction in astigmatism with suture removal (Figure 6-2).

Topographies are shown on June 16, August 4, September 1, and October 6. Note the nearly spherical results present on September 1 and on October 6. The larger spherical optical zone on October 6 resulted in a dramatic improvement in spectacle-corrected acuity. At this date, a refraction of -3.25 -1.50 x10 yielded 20/30 acuity.

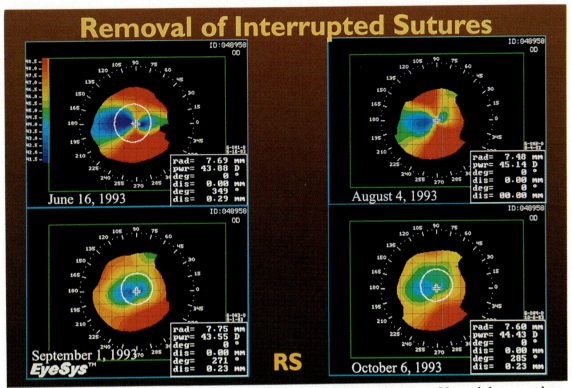

Figure 6-2. Progressive removal of multiple 10-0 Prolene interrupted sutures. Upper left image shows corneal appearance prior to suture removal. Lower right image shows corneal appearance after suture removal for reduction of astigmatism was completed.

Case 2: Management of Astigmatism with Sequential Suture Cutting

This 61 year-old female received penetrating keratoplasty for Fuch's dystrophy on the left eye on August 11, 1993. On September 13, irregular astigmatism caused best-corrected visual acuity of 20/200. Due to the corneal irregularity, an accurate refraction could not be obtained. Corneal topography on that date revealed a steep region inferonasally, so the suture at 195° was cut (Figure 6-3).

On October 4, refraction could not be obtained. The patient saw 20/400 uncorrected and 20/80 pinhole. Inferior steep regions observed on the topography contributed to corneal irregularity. Interrupted sutures at 210° and 330° were cut at this visit.

On October 18, surface irregularity and endothelial folds accounted for best-corrected visual acuity of 20/50. Refraction was -5.25 +2.00 x 103. Interrupted sutures at 135° and 285° were then cut. Four days later, refraction of -4.00 +0.50 x 50 yielded visual acuity of 20/50. There is still some corneal irregularity, and astigmatism management in this patient is ongoing.

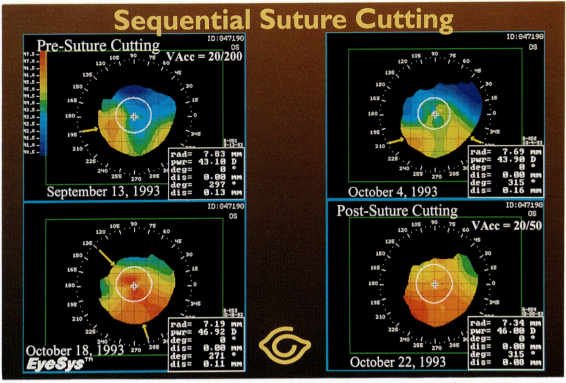

Figure 6-3. Sequential cutting of interrupted sutures. Upper left image shows corneal appearance prior to suture cut at 195° (arrow). Upper right image shows appearance prior to sutures cut at 210° and 330° (arrows). Lower left image, appearance prior to sutures cut at 135° and 285° (arrows). Lower right image, corneal appearance following the suture cutting. Corrected visual acuity has been improved from 20/200 to 20/50, although due to continuing corneal irregularity astigmatism management is ongoing.

Case 3: Reduction in Astigmatism Following Suture Cutting

This 75 year-old male status post penetrating keratoplasty for Fuch's dystrophy on the left eye on February 9, 1993 presented with regular astigmatism. Interrupted sutures at 45° and 225° were cut on March 8, 1993 (Figure 6-4A). One month later, the topographical change image reveals flattening in the steep meridian and steepening 90° away, although there is residual steepness nasally as seen in the upper right image taken April 12. Three interrupted sutures were then removed nasally, but due to the steepness of the cornea, radial keratotomy was performed on July 28. Figure 6-4B demonstrates the total effect of the suture cutting and RK. On August 23, refraction of -2.75 -0.75 x 45 yielded corrected acuity of 20/30. The topography demonstrates a relatively spherical cornea, with well-directed surgical effect.

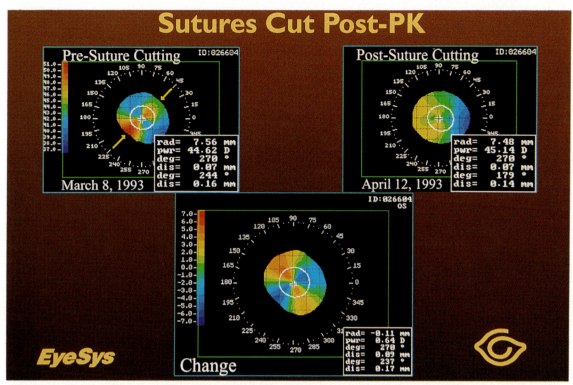

Figure 6-4A. Sutures cut at 45° and 225° (arrows). Upper left image shows appearance prior to suture cutting, upper right shows appearance one month later, and bottom image shows the induced changes to the corneal surface.

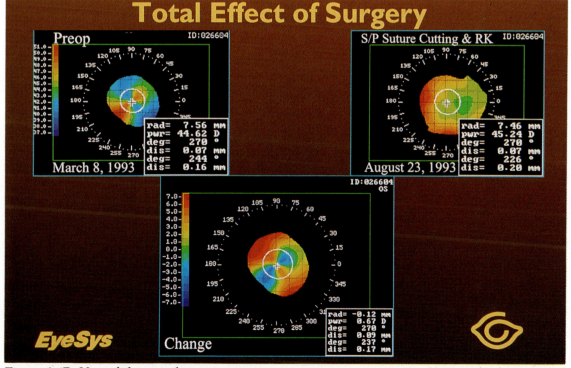

Figure 6-4B. Upper left image shows pre-astigmatism management appearance. Upper right shows corneal appearance following the cutting of five sutures and radial keratotomy. The bottom image shows the induced corneal changes caused by the combination of procedures.

Case 4: Adjustment of 24 Bite Running Suture with Reduction in Astigmatism

This 75 year-old female patient had Fuch's corneal dystrophy and decompensation following phacoemulsification with PC-IOL implantation elsewhere. She underwent penetrating kerato-plasty on July 8, 1993 in the left eye. On September 22, 1993, she announced that she was returning to Florida within one week and might not return. She desired suture adjustment to maximize her vision prior to departure, leading to the opportunity of performing multiple adjustments in one session and following them sequentially. Typically, only one, or occasionally two, adjustments are performed at a single session, and the graft is allowed to settle down in between suture adjustments. These progressive topographies illustrate the power of the suture adjustment guided by topography (Figure 6-5).

The first topography at 11:01 shows 5.64 D of astigmatism with a horizontal steep meridian. Refraction was +1.25 -6.00 x 110 yielding only 20/50 acuity. The suture was adjusted by tightening the sutures superiorly and inferiorly and feeding the material nasally and temporally, yielding the topography map at 13:46. Some degree of irregularity was nonetheless present, and a further adjustment in the suture was performed, tightening the suture material at 110° and moving it to the steepest hemi-meridian at 180°. This adjustment improved the sphericity in the superior area but accentuated the residual steep hemi-meridian at 290° as shown at 14:02. Further suture material was therefore tightened from the flattest hemi-meridian at 15° and moved to the steep hemi-meridian at 290°, yielding the topography at 14:15. Central topographic astigmatism remains slightly asymmetric but with a total 3-mm zone astigmatism of 1.05 D.

This case illustrates the power of suture adjustment to reduce suture-in astigmatism. As illustrated in Figure 6-5, the cornea may or may not remain stable when the sutures are later removed.[1]

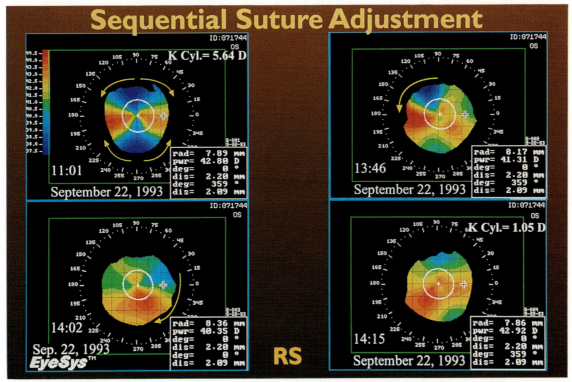

Figure 6-5. Sequential suture adjustment at a single visit. Upper left image shows corneal appearance prior to suture rotation. Loose suture material superiorly and inferiorly was fed nasally and temporally (arrows). Upper right, additional suture material superiorly was moved to 180° (arrow). Lower left, loose suture material at 15° was moved to 290° (arrow). Lower right, corneal appearance following suture rotation.

Case 5: Ineffectiveness of Wedge Resection Demonstrated

A 37 year-old female status post penetrating keratoplasty for keratoconus on August 1, 1983 in her left eye required hard contact lens correction for irregular astigmatism. However she had progressively poor contact lens tolerance due to difficulty of fit and topical allergies. The topography on December 2, 1992 (Figure 6-6) shows baseline astigmatism of over 9 D. Because of the excessive flattening inferotemporally, the wound was broken down in that area and resutured. On May 24, with three sutures still in place, partial return of the temporal flattening is seen, shifted superiorly. Dramatic further flattening had occurred with severely asymmetric astigmatism. The patient could not be refracted better than 20/100 and the remaining three sutures were removed. With all sutures removed, the wound appeared normal to clinical exam. Nevertheless the best refracted acuity was 20/200 with a refraction of 7.75 -5.00 x 170.

Accordingly, a wedge resection was performed on July 8, 1993. On September 8, after removal of the three tightest sutures, topography demonstrates less astigmatism, although steep in the area of the wedge resection. Asymmetry was still a factor. All sutures were removed at the time because the wound appeared well scarred two months postoperatively. The patient returned September 27. Even though the wound appeared secure, and over 1 mm of corneal tissue had been resected from the wound by the wedge resection, the overall topographic pattern and values bear a striking resemblance to the topography seen prior to the wedge resection (May 24).

This case illustrates the difficulty of dealing with some cases of post penetrating keratoplasty astigmatism. In particular, the ineffectiveness of wedge resections even with an apparently clinical stable wound is dramatically illustrated. It could be argued that impatience due to high degree of suture-in astigmatism led to premature suture removal, and that delaying suture removal longer would have yielded a better result. In the absence of frank wound separation, and in the presence of a good scar, however, it is unclear whether this was the case.

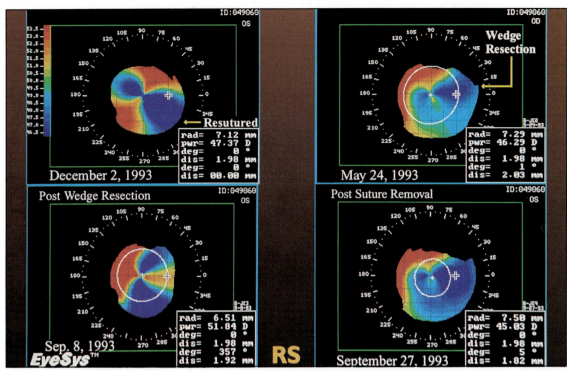

Figure 6-6. Resuturing of graft followed by wedge resection. Upper left, appearance prior to resuturing inferotemporally. Upper right, six months following resuturing. A wedge resection was performed temporally. Lower left, two months post wedge resection. All sutures were removed after this image was taken. Lower right, three weeks after sutures were removed, flattening has recurred in the location of the wedge resection.

Case 6: High Astigmatism after Loss of Running Suture, Repaired with Relaxing Incisions

This 80 year-old woman is status post penetrating keratoplasty with combined ECCE and PC-IOL in the left eye on November 10, 1990. Preoperative diagnosis was corneal scarring status post herpes zoster in the previous decade as well as previous cataract formation. Two years postoperatively with a 16 bite running 10-0 nylon suture and 8 interrupted 10-0 nylon sutures in place, acuity was stable with a refraction of +1.50 -4.25 x 155 yielding 20/30 vision. Six of the interrupted sutures were removed early postoperatively to reduce astigmatism, leaving the patient with the 16 bite running suture and two interrupted sutures (Figure 6-7). Topography showed symmetrical astigmatism consistent with the refraction (October 26, 1992). The patient presented with a broken running suture on July 20, 1993. The wound appeared well healed and the suture was removed in full. On August 10, she presented with two residual interrupted sutures and a refraction of +0.50 -4.75 x 135 yielding 20/30 acuity. The interrupted sutures were approximately in the orientation of the steep meridian and therefore were removed. On August 20 there was a slight increase in the asymmetry of the topography and the refraction was +3.00 -6.00 x 135 yielding 20/50 acuity. The patient was unhappy with this level of vision. She underwent relaxing incisions performed by breaking through the scar at Bowman's membrane and then separating the wound down to the level of Descemet's membrane. Approximately 60° incisions were performed in the steep hemi-meridians superotemporally and inferonasally guided by the topography.

The patient returned three weeks later. On October 6, 1993, marked reduction in the astigmatism, and some rotation of the residual astigmatism is seen. A refraction of +1.50 -2.00 x 175 yielded 20/30 acuity. The patient was pleased by the improvement in the quality of vision and accepted that refraction.

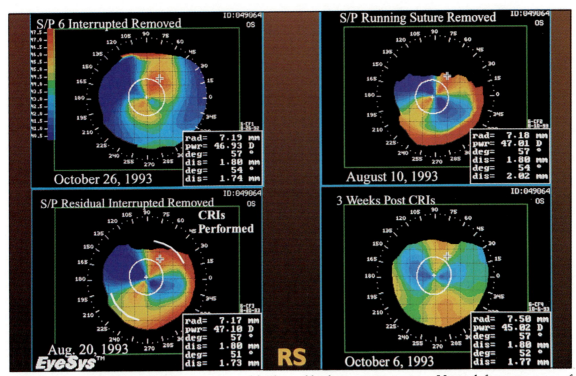

Figure 6-7. Correction of astigmatism caused by loss of broken running suture. Upper left, appearance of cornea with running suture in place. Six interrupted sutures had been removed early postoperatively. Upper right, appearance after broken running suture was removed. Lower left, appearance after the residual interrupted sutures were removed. Corneal relaxing incisions were performed at this visit. Lower right, three weeks following the relaxing incisions.

Reference

1. Filatov V, Steinert RF, Talamo JH: Postkeratoplasty astigmatism with single running suture or interrupted sutures. *Am J Ophth* 115:715-721, 1993.

7

Corneal Relaxing Incisions After Penetrating Keratoplasty

Johnny L. Gayton, MD
Spencer P. Thornton, MD, FACS

Introduction

The control of astigmatism induced by penetrating keratoplasty has been a most difficult challenge. The technique of corneal relaxing incisions has evolved over the past fourteen years since it was introduced by Troutman and Swinger[1] and is now the preferred method of reducing post-keratoplasty astigmatism.[2] It does not require sutures, gives rapid results, has a short postoperative course, and rarely gives overcorrection.

Current Management of Post-Keratoplasty Astigmatism

Penetrating keratoplasty has become increasingly successful with few serious complications, but high residual astigmatism still causes debilitating visual problems in these otherwise "successful" patients. Prior to the introduction of corneal relaxing incisions, which flatten the steeper meridian, the primary approach was the corneal wedge resection,[3] which steepened the flatter meridian. Relaxing incisions have been shown to be more predictable in effect, stable sooner after surgery, and less likely to produce overcorrections than wedge resection.[1,4-6]

As originally described, relaxing incisions were performed with a broken razor blade in a blade holder, with a gradually deepened incision under keratometric control to approximately one-third stromal depth at the slit lamp. The incisions were made approximately 60-80° of arc length, and, with one side done at a time, the procedure could be titrated by later adding another incision on the other side if needed.[1]

The following techniques are those which we have found useful in our hands.

Surgical Techniques

The Gayton Approach

In controlling postoperative astigmatism I aim at prevention as much as possible in the preoperative surgical plan. I generally make the graft 0.50 mm larger than the recipient bed. It is sutured into place with 8 interrupted sutures of 10-0 nylon. Nylon is easy to use and its color provides a contrast between it and the mersilene suture material used for the running suture, which is helpful in suture removal. The running suture is placed in a baseball stitch fashion with two bites being placed between each interrupted suture. At one month, or when the corneal edema resolves, whichever occurs later, I perform corneal topography. At that time, if there is an area of marked steepness, we will remove a nylon suture or sutures in the area or areas indicated by topography. I then have the patient return in two weeks for additional topography and further suture removal, if necessary. If simply removing sutures has taken care of most of the patient's astigmatism, we do not do anything else. However, if significant astigmatism persists, we will adjust the mersilene suture with jeweler's forceps. I have also used sterile jeweler's forceps to reopen the superficial aspect of the wound, allowing more flattening to occur.

If, despite suture and wound adjustment, the patient still has persistent visually disabling astigmatism, I perform relaxing incisions. The incisions are made with the Triple Edged Arcuate (TEA) blade. A 360° Thornton rule allows accurate measurement of the incision length.

I base the relaxing incisions on the corneal topography and perform them just anterior to the mersilene suture line. Corneal topography is essential in determining the proper length and location of these incisions. Keratometry readings and refraction can be deceptive, resulting in improper location of the incision. PK patients frequently have asymmetric astigmatism which can only be identified by topography.

The length of the incision in degrees is based on the patient's amount of astigmatism (as modified by the Thornton Nomogram) as well as the topographic picture. Since I have seen relatively wide separation of the incisions in some cases (Figures 7-1), I have elected to make the initial incisions at only 0.4-mm depth. If significant astigmatism persists postoperatively, I will deepen the incision if it has not demonstrated significant wound gape. If the incision gapes, I add another arcuate incision anterior to the previously placed incision. If possible, these incisions should be separated by 0.5 mm in order to prevent intersection of incisions.

I try to keep all astigmatic incisions in the graft in the unlikely event that a repeat corneal transplant is needed. This technique allows the patient to maintain a stable recipient bed. In patients who do not have a permanent suture in place, I will frequently perform the arcuate incisions in the graft-host interface, as I have found that they have more effect if placed in that

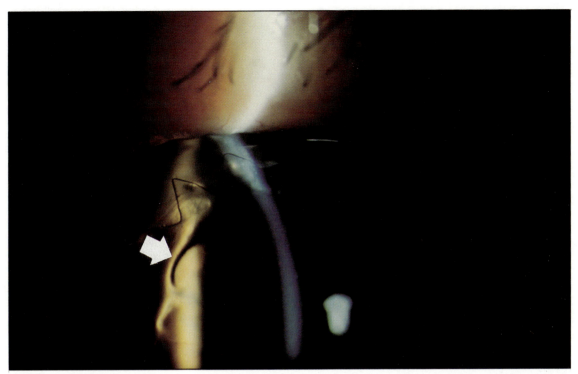

Figure 7-1. Wide separation (arrow) of corneal relaxing incision in a post penetrating keratoplasty patient.

location. Placing incisions in the graft-host interface must be done very carefully with accurate pachymetry in order to avoid perforation in a thin and weakened area. If additional incisions are needed, they are placed in the graft. If there are any questions about the integrity of the graft/host interface, all incisions should be placed anterior to the interface. We have found this technique to be most helpful in getting better postoperative visions more quickly in our corneal transplant patients.

If, in addition to the astigmatism, the post-graft patient has significant disabling myopia, I perform an RK procedure in the corneal graft. The incisions are made "American" style and stop just anterior to the mersilene suture or the graft-host interface. I have found that it is best to correct the myopia prior to making any astigmatic incisions. In some cases, simply flattening the central cornea with radial incisions will also decrease a patient's astigmatism significantly. In other cases, the astigmatism will actually increase. I wait until the corneal topography is stable before making any astigmatic incision following radial incisions.

The Thornton Approach

I use a triple-edged diamond blade on a micrometer handle (Figure 7-2) to make all corneal incisions in correcting astigmatism, and measure the length of my incisions in degrees of arc as determined by a 360° ruler (Figure 7-3) which is printed on the cornea just prior to the placement of incisions. I base the length of my incisions on the amount of astigmatism as modified by age and other modifiers in my nomogram, and rely greatly on the information provided by EyeSys

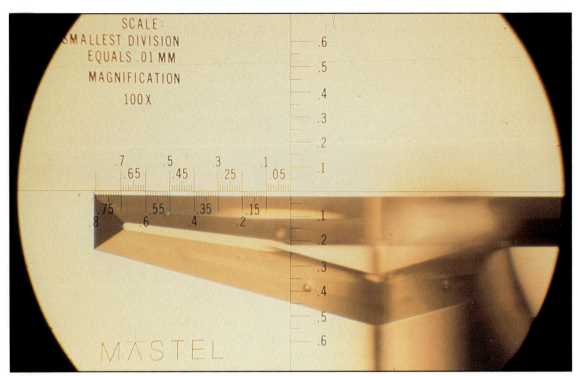

Figure 7-2. Thornton triple-edged arcuate diamond blade.

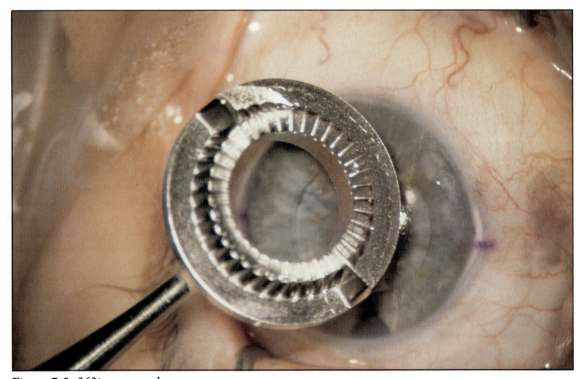

Figure 7-3. 360° arcuate ruler.

topography. With the information provided by topography I have been able to identify asymmetric and non-orthogonal astigmatism as well as identify the width of the steep areas more accurately than with keratometry or any other diagnostic means. This ability has allowed a refinement of technique that has included asymmetric incisions, single-sided incisions, straight, arcuate, and inverse arcuate incisions for greater surgical control and predictability.

Rather than use shallower incisions to avoid uncontrolled wound gape, I use shorter incisions, placed 98% deep. I have not seen a problem with wound gape with this approach, and when higher degrees of correction are desired, I use additional pairs of incisions inside the outer incisions, with all incisions placed inside the graft-host interface. If I am using a single pair of arcuate incisions I place them at the 7-mm optical zone, and if two or more pairs of incisions are required I place the outer pair just inside the graft-host interface at the 8-mm optical zone.

Relaxing incisions are relatively easy to perform with the new instruments available and result in faster visual recovery than the technically more complex wedge resection. Relaxing incisions alone are my procedure of choice in post-keratoplasty astigmatism of less than 10 D.

Corneal Topography of Corneal Relaxing Incisions in Post-Keratoplasty Patients

Figure 7-4 demonstrates corneal topography of a 30 year-old male who received penetrating keratoplasty for keratoconus in the right eye in 1982. He presented in December, 1992 with 7.5 D of myopia and 5.25 D of keratometric cylinder. Eight incision radial keratotomy was performed at the 3.5-mm optical zone, as well as two arcuate corneal relaxing incisions of 30° of arc at 0.56-mm depth at the 6 and 8-mm optical zones. Since the preoperative topography demonstrated asymmetrical inferonasal steepness, the CRIs were both placed at axis 330°.

The six month postoperative image indicates rotation of the astigmatism, but the change image demonstrates successful flattening in the meridian of the CRIs. Since radial incisions were placed, there is no coupling evident, that is, no steepening 90° away from the CRIs.

Two weeks later, two additional CRIs of 50° of arc were performed at the graft/host interface at 0.4-mm depth to treat 4.63 D of residual astigmatism (Figure 7-5). The six week postoperative topographic image demonstrates a more spherical central cornea. Since no radials were performed in conjunction with these CRIs, the change image shows coupling, with flattening in the incision meridian and steepening 90° away.

Figure 7-6 demonstrates the total effect of the surgeries. Almost 5 D of flattening was induced in the formerly steep inferonasal region. The patient's uncorrected vision has gone from finger count to 20/80$^+$ and final refraction is -2.75 +1.50 x 80.

Figure 7-7 shows the topography of a 72 year-old male who underwent penetrating keratoplasty in the left eye for Fuch's dystrophy in 1988. By 1990, all sutures had been removed. Three years later, the patient presented with significant myopia and astigmatism. Refraction was -12.75 +5.50 x 64. Keratometry found 4 D of cylinder at 63°.

Corneal topography revealed asymmetric steepness superiorly which extended into the visual axis. Accordingly, eight radial incisions at the 3-mm optical zone were performed in addition to a superiorly placed relaxing incision at the graft/host interface, 60° of arc.

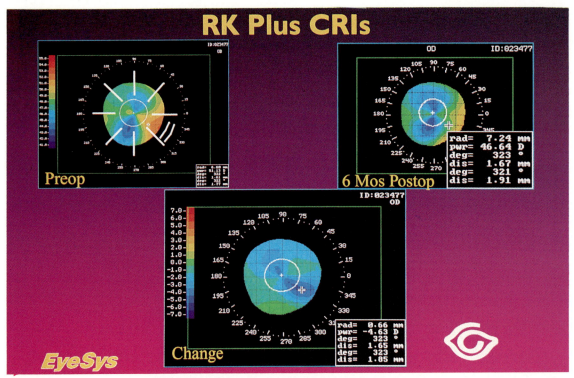

Figure 7-4. Corneal topography of a post penetrating keratoplasty case who received 8-incision radial keratotomy and two arcuate relaxing incisions inferonasally. Upper left image—preoperative corneal appearance, upper right image—appearance six months postoperatively, bottom image—surgically induced corneal change.

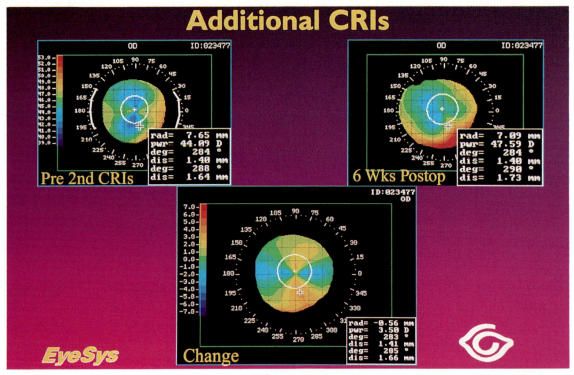

Figure 7-5. Same patient in Figure 7-4. Upper left image—corneal appearance prior to additional corneal relaxing incisions at graft/host interface, upper right image—corneal appearance six weeks following the second pair of CRIs, bottom image—surgically induced change.

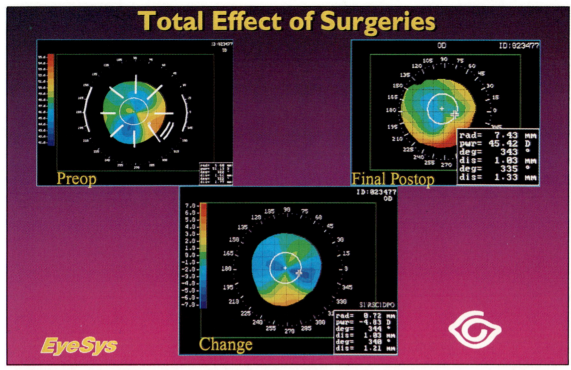

Figure 7-6. Same patient in Figures 7-4 and 7-5. Upper left image—corneal appearance prior to refractive surgeries, upper right image—corneal appearance following refractive surgeries, bottom image, total surgically induced changes.

The topographic change image demonstrates the effect of the combined surgeries. There is marked flattening in the meridian of the CRI, but due to the radials there is no steepening 90° away. Although the postoperative image still demonstrates superior steepening, the steep region is more peripheral. Keratometry found only 1.72 D of cylinder. Final refraction is -3.00 +0.75 x 115.

Figure 7-8 displays topography of a 34 year-old female who received penetrating keratoplasty in both eyes in 1988 for keratoconus. On February 22, 1993, CRIs were performed on the right eye. Preoperatively the refraction was -1.75 +2.25 x 125 with 3 D of keratometric cylinder. Corneal topography determined placement of the incisions. Two incisions were made at the graft/host interface at 0.6-mm depth, each 40° of arc.

Postoperatively the refraction was -1.00 sph, and keratometry was 41.87/42 x 84. Topography demonstrated flattening in the incision meridian and steepening 90° away. The postoperative image indicates a breakup of the astigmatism pattern with a nearly spherical central cornea.

After the successful result in the right eye, CRIs were performed on the left eye (Figure 7-9). These incisions were also placed at the graft/host interface at 0.6 mm depth. A longer arcuate incision was placed nasally because of asymmetry of astigmatism as determined by topography.

The surgery resulted in an overcorrection, which progressed later postoperatively. At three months, a pair of CRIs was performed at the graft/host interface to counteract the overcorrection. Because of the strong response to the first pair of CRIs, this pair was initially made at 0.4 mm depth. These incisions mildly reduced the overcorrection, but the effect regressed. The incisions

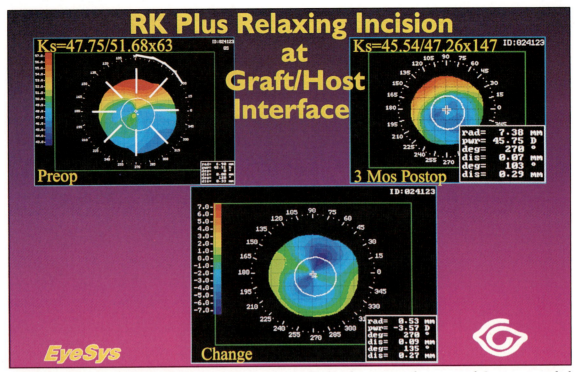

Figure 7-7. Corneal topography of a post penetrating keratoplasty case who received 8-incision radial keratotomy and a superior corneal relaxing incision at the graft/host interface.

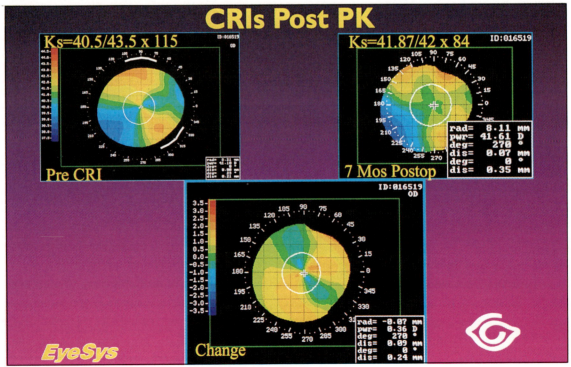

Figure 7-8. Topography of a post penetrating keratoplasty case who received two arcuate relaxing incisions at the graft/host interface placed at the areas of greatest corneal steepness as determined by preoperative corneal topography.

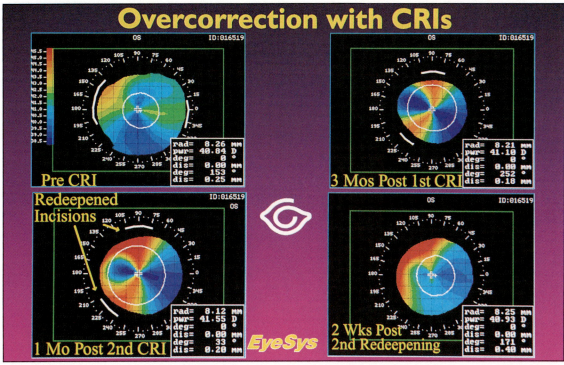

Figure 7-9. Fellow eye of patient shown in Figure 7-8. A pair of arcuate relaxing incisions made at a depth of 0.6 mm at the graft/host interface (upper left) caused severe overcorrection (upper right). An additional pair of CRIs were placed to counteract the overcorrection at the graft/host interface at a depth of 0.4 mm. The lower left image illustrates the corneal appearance following the second pair of CRIs. The lower right image shows the appearance after these CRIs were redeepened twice to a total depth of 0.6 mm.

were deepened to 0.5 mm depth, but the patient still complained of poor vision in the left eye and difficulty driving at night. The incisions were deepened again to 0.6 mm depth. Following the second redeepening, the keratometry was 39.75/43 x 89. Topography indicated a more spherical central cornea, although peripheral superonasal steepness persists. This case demonstrates the variability in reaction to CRIs among graft cases. Unlike refractive surgery in other types of patients, individual variability is not the factor. The tension of the donor button probably accounts for most of the variability. In this patient the right eye had an excellent result. However, greater tension on the donor button on the left eye caused dramatically greater effect of the CRIs. The cornea likely pulled at these incisions, which would account for the progression of effect. To avoid this problem, the surgeon (JLG) now uses incisions at 0.4 mm depth and deepens them later if more effect is desired.

Figure 7-10 displays the topography of a patient's right eye status post penetrating keratoplasty in 1982. The patient required a hard contact lens for good acuity but progressive contact lens intolerance limited wearing time in the right eye.

Evaluation disclosed a refraction of -1.50 -6.00 x 155 yielding 20/30 acuity. Topography showed over 6 D of central astigmatism with a moderately regular pattern. Arcuate keratotomy was performed with a 6.0-mm optical zone centered on the visual axis. Each incision was 75° in length. Incisions were centered on the 70° meridian as indicated by topography.

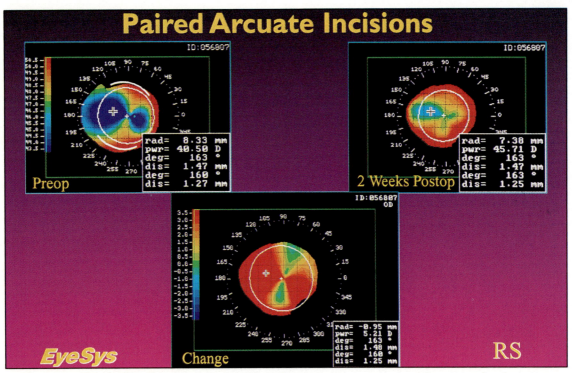

Figure 7-10. Topography of post penetrating keratoplasty case receiving a pair of arcuate relaxing incisions. The change image (bottom) indicates significant coupling, that is, steepening 90° away from the incisions (Courtesy of Roger Steinert, MD).

Follow-up examination two weeks postoperatively showed dramatic change in the topography. Central astigmatism was less than 1 D, with mild asymmetry. It is interesting to note that the originally flatter hemi-meridian temporally at approximately 170° persists. Refraction was -4.00 -1.50 x 150 yielding 20/25 acuity. Interestingly, the change image demonstrates little flattening in the incision meridian, but significant steepening 90° away.

Figure 7-11 displays topography of a 28 year-old female with a history of bilateral retinitis pigmentosa and herpetic keratitis in the left eye who required penetrating keratoplasty in 1981, and because of recurrent herpetic keratitis had to have a second penetrating keratoplasty in 1984. Recurrences since then have been controlled with Viroptic, but vision has been poor. The preoperative examination showed best-corrected vision of 20/50⁻ with a refraction of -9.50 + 6.25 x 135. Surgery was deferred because of recent herpetic keratitis, but due to severe astigmatic anisometropia she requested astigmatism reduction surgery. On re-examination seven months later, her best-corrected vision was still 20/50⁻. The 8-mm graft button was noted to be fairly clear and non-reactive. Keratometry was 43.37/50.75 x 133, and uncorrected vision was 20/200.

Three pairs of CRIs were performed in conjunction with four radials to reduce the myopia to near the level of her right eye (-0.50 -2.75 x 175, VAcc = 20/30). One week postoperatively, refraction was +0.75 -1.25 x 50 with 20/30⁻ best-corrected visual acuity. At her latest visit, six months postoperatively, she had 3.75 D of residual keratometric cylinder, 20/60 uncorrected vision, and 20/30⁻ corrected vision.

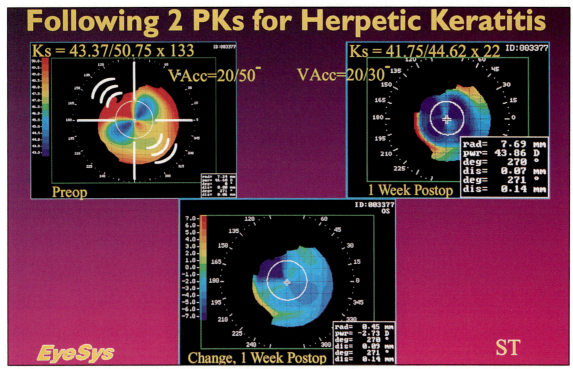

Figure 7-11. Topography of post penetrating keratoplasty case receiving 4-incision radial keratotomy and three pairs of arcuate incisions within the donor button.

Figure 7-12 shows topography of a 75 year-old female four years post penetrating keratoplasty and 12 years post cataract and IOL surgery OD. Preoperatively, the refraction was -4.50 +6.25 x 25 with best-corrected visual acuity of 20/70. Because topography revealed asymmetry in astigmatism, two 50° arcuate incisions were placed across the 35° semi-meridian superiorly and one 50° arcuate incision was placed across the 215° semi-meridian inferiorly. The arcuate incisions were kept within the graft button.

Figure 7-12A compares the preoperative and two-week postoperative topographical appearance. The change graph demonstrates the marked flattening in the incision meridian with steepening 90° away. At three months postoperatively (Figure 7-12B), the coupling has regressed, leaving only the flattening in the incision meridian. Although there is residual keratometric cylinder, refraction is -0.75 -0.50 x 85 and the best-corrected visual acuity has improved to 20/25.

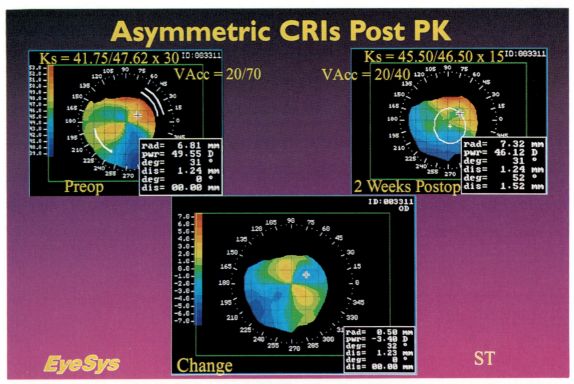

Figure 7-12A. Two week postoperative topography. The change image (bottom) indicates flattening in the incision meridian with coupling, that is, steepening 90° away.

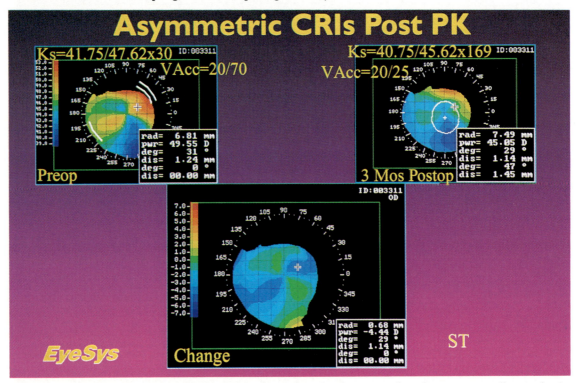

Figure 7-12B. Three month postoperative topography. As shown in the change image (bottom), the flattening persists, but the coupling has regressed.

Figure 7-12. Topography of post penetrating keratoplasty case receiving two relaxing incisions superonasally and one inferotemporally within the donor button.

References

1. Troutman RC, Swinger C: Relaxing incisions for control of postoperative astigmatism following keratoplasty. *Ophthalmic Surgery* 11:117-120, 1980.

2. Thornton SP, Sanders DR: Graded nonintersecting transverse incisions for correction of idiopathic astigmatism. *J Cataract Refract Surg* 13:27-31, 1987.

3. Troutman RC: Microsurgical control of corneal astigmatism in cataract and keratoplasty. *Tram Acad Ophth & Otol* 77:563-572, 1973.

4. Krachmer JH, Fenzl RE: Surgical correction of high postkeratoplasty astigmatism. *Arch Ophthalmol* 98:1400-1402, 1980.

5. Sugar J, Kirk AK: Relaxing keratotomy for post-keratoplasty high astigmatism. *Ophthalmic Surg* 14:156-158, 1983.

6. Lavery GW, Lindstrom RL, Hofer LA, Doughman DJ: The surgical management of corneal astigmatism after penetrating keratoplasty. *Ophthalmic Surg* 16:165-169, 1985.

8

Corneal Transplantation and Astigmatic Keratotomy

ROBERT G. MARTIN, MD

Introduction

The treatment of corneal astigmatism in a corneal graft is more complex and frustrating than in almost any ocular condition. Thus, it is far better to try to prevent corneal astigmatism in corneal transplantation. However, in spite of running suture adjustment, selective suture removal, suction trephines, and automated trephines, too many corneal transplants are left with astigmatism that is not correctable with contact lenses or glasses. These and other methods have, however, helped to reduce astigmatism in a larger percentage of patients. Hopefully future techniques and technology will help even further in reducing this visually disabling disorder so that surgical treatment is not necessary.

I have been developing my techniques for controlling astigmatism in corneal grafts with astigmatic keratotomy (AK) since the mid 1970s, and I am still learning. No one has the final answer on treating astigmatism in these patients; indeed, most studies on this subject, in my experience, have been flawed because of lack of standardized parameters and techniques, non-randomization of cases, and even lack of experience. As in all teachings on techniques, instrumentation and nomograms, it is important to use the errors of the instructors and what they have learned as a starting point for you, the individual surgeon, to decrease your complications and improve the technique in your hands. The surgical technique that I am doing today involves far less surgery with much more efficacy and predictability than what I was doing in the mid '70s through the '80s.

In spite of new technology such as the micron diamond knife, the micron scope, intraoperative corneoscopes or keratometer, and intraoperative pachymetry, astigmatic keratotomy is still less predictable in corneal grafts than in post-cataract, intraoperative cataract, and primary astigmatic cases. Technology is, however, enabling us to better evaluate these cases, leading us toward more predictable outcomes. The advent of corneal topography has given us one of the best tools to define the preoperative condition, allowing us to better direct our surgery, and to evaluate the effect of the surgical procedure, that is, outcome.

One problem affecting predictability in graft cases is the variable thickness of the corneal tissue, which most nomograms do not take into account. With a corneal graft the cornea 1/2 or 1/4 mm from the incision site can have a significantly different corneal thickness. It is important for the operative surgeon to measure intraoperatively the pachymetry on the site of the astigmatism where the incision will be placed, and choose an incision site where the corneal thickness is not variable.

Making incisions in the patient's recipient corneal tissue or in the wound has proven, in my hands, to be very ineffective in correcting corneal astigmatism and I would discourage it. Using a 7-mm optical zone on a 7.75-mm donor button almost always creates a situation where corneal depth varies so much over the 2-mm length of the incision that the correction is unpredictable. Corneal relaxing incisions (CRIs) work best on the donor tissue at a point where the thickness of the cornea is rather standard over the area of the incision.

Indications and Contraindications for AK

Indications

1. Patients with stable corneal topography, showing no change in the change map.
2. Stable refraction.
3. Patients who have a need to have a better quality of vision without glasses or contact lens.
4. A patient who cannot function without contacts or glasses to comfortably correct their refractive error. If a significant anisometropia has been induced in addition to corneal astigmatism, combining radial keratotomy with the astigmatism can be helpful.

Contraindications

1. The patient who functions well without glasses, with glasses, or with a contact lens.
2. A patient whose refraction has not stabilized, documented on two 3-month illustrations using corneal topography and refraction to make sure the refraction and the shape of the cornea is stable. Change maps with corneal topography are very helpful. Figure 8-1 demonstrates a case where the shape of the cornea is not yet stable.
3. A patient with corneal edema or graft rejection.

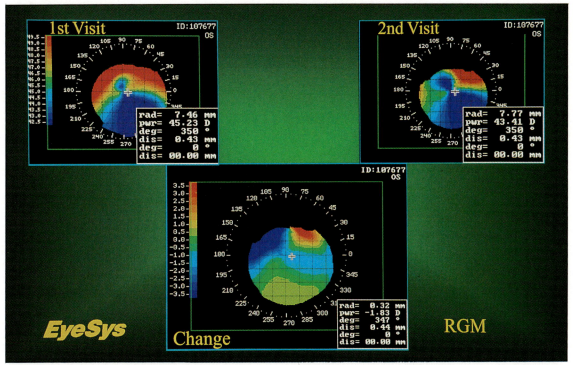

Figure 8-1. Corneal topography of two visits post penetrating keratoplasty. The difference map (bottom), taken by subtracting the data points of the second visit from the first, demonstrates corneal changes, indicating that the cornea is not stable.

4. A patient with blepharitis or infection which is not controlled.

5. A patient who refuses surgery.

Technique

The technique of corneal relaxing incisions in this group mirrors the technique that I am now doing on postoperative or intraoperative patients with cataract extraction and intraocular lens implantation, which is fully described in Chapter 3. However there are some differences in graft cases and particular aspects of the technique that should be emphasized. First refractions, keratometric readings, and, most importantly, corneal topography change images must be stable.

The topography is used as a map to determine where to place the astigmatic keratotomy incisions. The plus axis of astigmatism is marked at the limbus and on the cornea near the graft/donor junction using a standard surgical marking pencil (Figure 8-2). After the marks are done the surgery should be performed within forty-five minutes to avoid dissipation of the marks.

Usually a 7-mm marker is used to mark around the central visual axis. However the incision(s) are rarely placed at this zone because intraoperative pachymetry is performed next and usually the readings are so variable near the graft/donor recipient edge that it is necessary to move

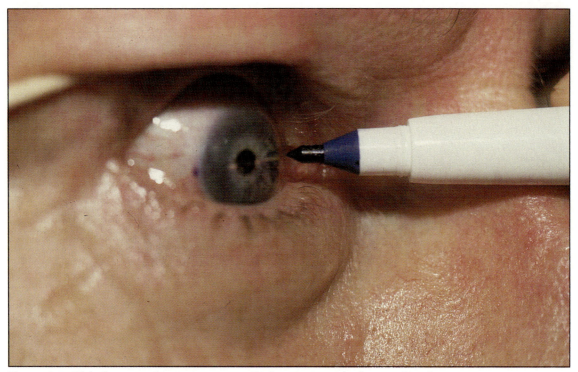

Figure 8-2. The plus axis of astigmatism is marked using a standard surgical marking pen.

in about 0.50 to 1 mm on each side before there are consistent readings over the length of the incisions. Thus, most of these incisions are made at about the 6.50-mm optical zone on a 7.75-mm graft. The intraoperative pachymetry probe is used to measure on exactly the point to be incised. As a rule of thumb, approximately 3 D of effect per mm incision at full thickness depth will be achieved if the incisions are greater than, or equal to, 1.5 mm. Keeping these incisions less than 45° of arc is important.

Try to avoid perforating. Thus you might want to pull back 10-15 microns from 100% depth to avoid perforation. In making a 2-mm incision, measure with pachymetry at either side of the 2-mm incision because depths can change. An alternative technique to using intraoperative pachymetry is to use corneal spreaders, spread, and cut down to Descemet's membrane so that there is always the same depth of incision.

After one incision is made, and frequently one incision is all that is needed (it is not unusual to achieve 6 D of correction with one 3-mm or 2.5-mm incision), take the pressure off the globe, and remeasure with the intraoperative corneoscope, although be aware that measurements with the corneoscope, in my experience, can be very misleading. If there is a significant correction, but the full astigmatism is not quite corrected, consider doing no additional surgery. Instead re-evaluate the result postoperatively to determine if more correction is needed. The most common error is overcorrecting. With two 3-mm CRIs, I have achieved 20 or more diopters of correction in patients who needed only 10 D of correction using this technique. It is better to undercorrect and make the patient better and then determine if more is needed at a later date.

Following these corneal transplant cases postoperatively requires much more diligence than in other patients. Incising the cornea can encourage graft rejection and/or infection. Perforating the cornea gives much more correction. If a perforation occurs on the first incision and the original surgery plan called for two incisions, I would encourage you to hold off, evaluate the result and when it stabilizes, if additional correction is needed, then consider adding another incision at a later date.

In 98% of the CRIs in corneal grafts that I have performed, two or fewer incisions are required; in 50% of the graft cases who need astigmatism correction, only one incision is required. Remember it is always better to undercorrect than overcorrect. You can always add an incision if the cornea is undercorrected, but if you end up overcorrecting, you will find that you have to add another set of incisions, usually at right angles to the original incision(s). In my experience, if you keep chasing the astigmatism around the eye, you can induce the myopia of a hexagonal keratotomy type incision. Postoperatively, follow these patients closely, and have them come in within twenty-four hours at any sign of reduced vision, increased foreign body sensation or ocular redness. Cover them with antibiotics topically as long as the incision is not re-epithelialized. In spite of cautions against using antibiotic ointment, I often apply polysporin ointment or another broad spectrum antibiotic ointment to the lid margins h.s. in addition to topical anti-inflammatory drugs such as Tobrex, Ciloxan or Ocuflox.

Nomogram

Graft cases experience about three times as much correction as other patients. About 1.5 to 2 D of effect are achieved in these cases per millimeter of incision length at 95 to 100% depth. Each cut should be a minimum of 1.5 mm and a maximum of 3.5 mm. All incisions should be arcuate. Avoid performing incisions at less than the 5-mm optical zone.

Topographical Case Studies

Figure 8-3 shows topography of a 30 year-old woman who had penetrating keratoplasty in 1992 for corneal leukoma and severe keratoconus. Six months later she received a pair of relaxing incisions to correct 9 D of refractive cylinder. Since topography indicated greater steepness inferiorly, the inferior CRI was made slightly longer than the superior (3 mm versus 2 mm).

The surgery reduced the refractive cylinder by more than half. Three months postoperatively the refraction was -5.0 +4.0 x 89. The change image indicates that about 2 D of flattening occurred in the incision meridian and about 3.75 D of steepening occurred 90° away.

Figure 8-4 shows the topography of a 72 year-old woman who had extracapsular cataract extraction, and penetrating keratoplasty for decompensated bullous keratopathy. Ten months later she received a single 3-mm arcuate relaxing incision to correct 8 D of refractive cylinder.

The topographic change image demonstrates the tremendous effect of the relaxing incision. In addition to flattening in the incision meridian, over 7 D of steepening occurred 90° away. Five months postoperatively the refraction is +1.00 +0.50 x 33. Thus 7.5 D reduction of astigmatism was achieved with 3 mm of incision length, or over 2 D of effect per mm.

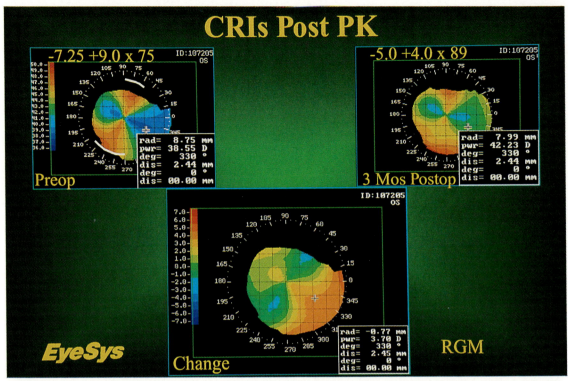

Figure 8-3. Topography of case receiving a pair of CRIs post penetrating keratoplasty. The inferior CRI was 3 mm long, and the superior CRI was 2 mm long. Upper left shows preoperative corneal appearance, upper right shows three months postoperative appearance, and bottom shows surgically induced changes.

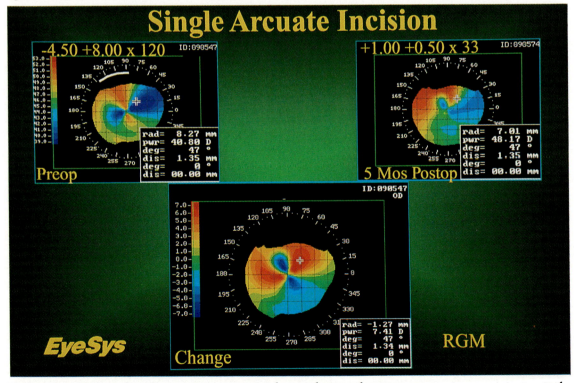

Figure 8-4. Topography of case post penetrating keratoplasty and cataract extraction receiving a single 3-mm superior relaxing incision. Upper left shows preoperative corneal appearance, upper right shows three months postoperative appearance, and bottom shows surgically induced changes.

Shown in Figure 8-5 is the topography of a 77 year-old woman who received penetrating keratoplasty for bullous keratopathy. Nine months later she received a single 2-mm arcuate relaxing incision to correct superotemporal steepness. Preoperatively, her refraction was -3.50 +7.25 x 39, with 20/40 corrected acuity and 20/150 uncorrected acuity. Three weeks following the procedure, as shown in the topography, her refraction was -2.00 +3.00 x 79, with 20/50 corrected acuity and 20/80 uncorrected acuity. The change image (bottom) illustrates the flattening induced at the incision site and the steepening induced 90° away. The last available refraction, taken one month later, is -1.50 +1.75 x 80, with 20/40 corrected vision and 20/40 uncorrected vision.

Figure 8-6 shows topography of an 80 year-old man aphakic in the left eye who received penetrating keratoplasty for Fuch's dystrophy, and secondary IOL implantation in 1988. Four pairs of relaxing incisions were performed in 1989. In October, 1993 he received 4-incision radial keratotomy and two 2.4-mm arcuate corneal relaxing incisions at the areas of greatest steepness. Preoperatively the refraction was -13.25 +12.00 x 52 with a best corrected visual acuity of 20/50[+1] and uncorrected vision of 20/200. One week postoperatively the refraction was -5.25 +5.75 x 65 with corrected acuity of 20/30[-2] and uncorrected acuity of 20/60. The patient is happy with his refraction, as now he is able to read without glasses.

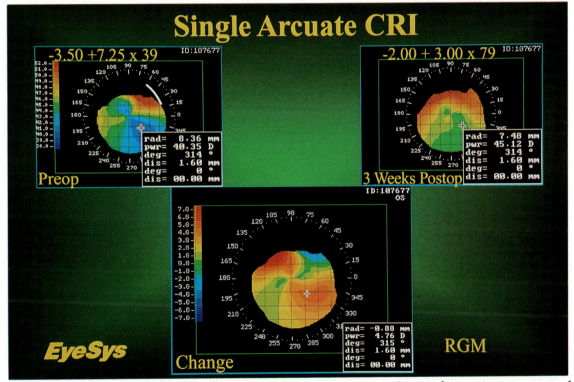

Figure 8-5. Topography of post penetrating keratoplasty case receiving a 2-mm relaxing incision at area of greatest steepness. Upper left shows preoperative corneal appearance, upper right shows three months postoperative appearance, and bottom shows surgically induced changes.

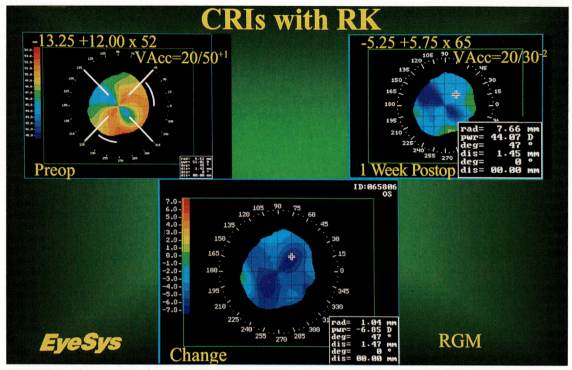

Figure 8-6. Topography of case post penetrating keratoplasty and secondary IOL implantation, and post previous astigmatic keratotomy, receiving 4-incision radial keratotomy and two 2.4-mm relaxing incisions. Upper left shows preoperative corneal appearance, upper right shows three months postoperative appearance, and bottom shows surgically induced changes.

The patient illustrated in Figure 8-7, an 80 year-old female, received cataract extraction and CRIs five months following penetrating keratoplasty for bullous keratopathy. She received a single 1.5-mm relaxing incision at axis 135° to correct severe superior steepness.

Preoperatively, she had 4.5 D of keratometric cylinder and 20/100 uncorrected vision. Two months postoperatively, the axis of astigmatism shifted, but the superior steepness persisted. She still had 20/100 uncorrected vision and 4.37 D of keratometric cylinder at 96° at that visit. At four months postoperatively, the refraction was -4.75 + 5.75 x 96. Another relaxing incision 1.5 mm in length was performed at 96°. One day following the enhancement, the astigmatism was markedly reduced. The refraction was -1.75 + 2.75 x 75, with 20/30⁻ best-corrected acuity. Although there was still corneal irregularity, with superonasal steepness and inferotemporal flatness, the patient achieved 20/40 uncorrected acuity.

Figure 8-8 shows topography of a 64 year-old woman who had penetrating keratoplasty in 1992. One year later she received 4-incision radial keratotomy at a 4.75-mm optical zone and a single CRI to correct 4.25 D of myopia and 3.5 D of astigmatism. Four months postoperatively the refraction was -3.25 + 1.00 x 45, with 20/30 corrected acuity and 20/100⁺ uncorrected acuity.

Five months postoperatively the radial keratotomy was enhanced by reducing the optical zone to 4.25 mm. Prior to enhancement, the refraction was -3.75 + 1.50 x 55. One week following the enhancement the refraction was -1.25 + 1.00 x 15, with 20/30⁻ best-corrected, as well as

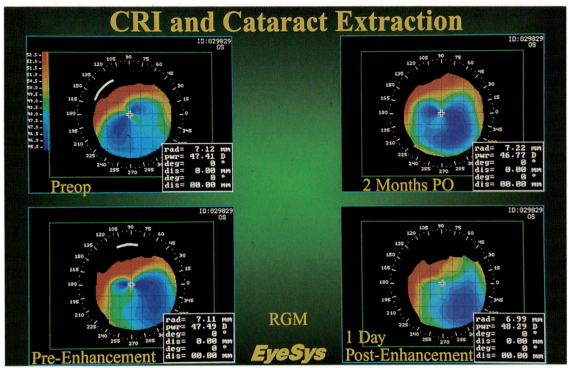

Figure 8-7. Topography of case post penetrating keratoplasty receiving cataract extraction and a 1.5-mm superior relaxing incision. Upper left shows preoperative appearance, upper right shows two month postoperative appearance, bottom left shows four month postoperative appearance. At the four month visit, a second 1.5-mm superior relaxing incision was performed. The bottom right image shows one day following the enhancement.

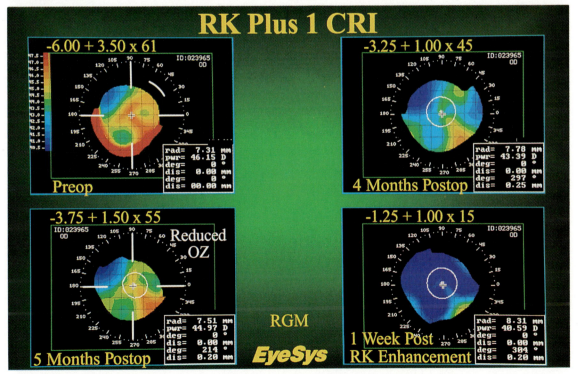

Figure 8-8. Topography of post penetrating case receiving 4-incision radial keratotomy at the 4.75-mm optical zone and a single CRI. Upper left shows the preoperative appearance and upper right shows the four month postoperative appearance. Bottom left shows the five month postoperative appearance. At this visit, the radial keratotomy optical zone was reduced to 4.25 mm. Bottom right shows the corneal appearance one week following the enhancement.

uncorrected, visual acuity. The lower right image on the topography demonstrates the flattening achieved by the enhancement.

Figure 8-9 shows topography of a 56 year-old man who had penetrating keratoplasty in 1954. In 1983 he presented with cataract and 5 D of keratometric cylinder at 102°. The preoperative topography indicated inferior steepness, so a single 3-mm relaxing incision at the 7-mm optical zone was performed at the time of the cataract extraction.

The upper right image in the topography indicates a large overcorrection caused by the incision. The cornea was very distorted, so keratometry could not be performed. Refraction indicated -5.25 +11.50 x 7, with 20/60 best-corrected vision. The incision site was debrided and sutured, in an attempted to reduce the overcorrection.

Two months following the suturing, the refraction was -2.50 +6.00 x 5, with 20/50 best-corrected vision. At this time, an additional relaxing incision was performed temporally to reduce the overcorrection further. Two months following this incision, the refraction was -3.25 +3.75 x 180, with 20/50 best-corrected vision. Astigmatism management is still ongoing in this patient.

This example illustrates the variability of response that should be expected in penetrating keratoplasty cases. This patient had 3 to 4 D of effect per mm of incision, which is about twice the average. It is unknown what caused this tremendous surgical effect, although the long time elapsed since corneal transplantation (almost 30 years) may have been a factor.

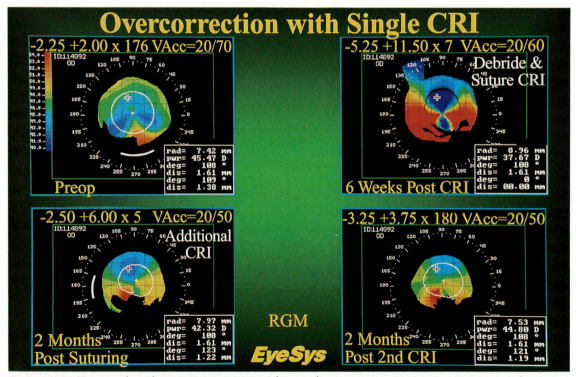

Figure 8-9. Topography of case post penetrating keratoplasty receiving cataract extraction and a 3-mm inferior relaxing incision. Upper left shows the preoperative corneal appearance and the upper right shows the six week postoperative appearance, indicating large overcorrection. At this visit the CRI was debrided and sutured. The lower left image shows corneal appearance two months later. At this visit a temporal relaxing incision was performed. The lower right image shows appearance two months later.

Discussion

In general, surgeons should expect less predictability in penetrating keratoplasty cases, as there are factors, such as the length of time the donor cornea has been in place, variable thickness, and tension on the corneal button, that cannot be controlled for in present nomograms. Surgeons should aim for undercorrection in these cases, and enhance if necessary. It is far better to undercorrect than to chase astigmatism around the eye. If a cautious approach is taken in these patients, visually disabling astigmatism can be substantially reduced in the vast majority of cases.

Section III

Wound Management Techniques in Cataract Surgery

9

Cataract Incisions at the Steep Axis

Johnny L. Gayton, MD
Patrick Rowan, MD
Michelle A. Van Der Karr

Introduction

Before the advent of small-incision cataract surgery, surgeons were more concerned with techniques to reduce the large astigmatism induced by the incision and sutures than with correcting pre-existing astigmatism. However, as incisions were reduced from 12 to 14 mm to 6 to 7 mm, the amount of astigmatism induced by the incision became more predictable. Some surgeons began using the induced astigmatism to counteract the pre-existing astigmatism.

With sutured, superior cataract incisions, wound manipulation techniques involved altering suture tension and wound architecture.[1-3] For with-the-rule astigmatism, the wound was created more shallow so that it would slip somewhat postoperatively, and the sutures were fewer and looser so as not to cause tension. These incisions would then flatten the cornea in the vertical meridian. For against-the-rule astigmatism, the wound was created deeper, and more sutures were used with greater tension. These incisions would then steepen the cornea in the vertical meridian.

With sutureless incisions, there is no opportunity for correcting astigmatism by using a tighter wound. The sutureless incision can only be made relatively astigmatically neutral or made to slip so that it will flatten the cornea in the incision meridian. Thus against-the-rule astigmatism cannot be corrected by a superior sutureless incision.

New wound manipulation techniques involve flattening the steep axis with the cataract incision. This strategy involves rotating the incision to the steep axis. Although moving the incision requires considerable adjustments in the operating room, once the change to a new position is mastered, operating temporally or obliquely is actually quite easy.

The Gayton Approach

Patients having with-the-rule astigmatism are generally well served by current top-approach sutureless cataract techniques. However, against-the-rule astigmatism frequently is worsened by a superiorly placed cataract incision. The goal with the Gayton approach, which has been developed with the experience of 7,000 rotated cases, is to ensure that at the very least against-the-rule astigmatism is not worsened, and at best somewhat reduced.

Sutureless scleral-tunnel incisions which are designed to slip somewhat are placed at the steep axis of astigmatism, either 6 or 7 mm in length depending on the amount of preoperative astigmatism. In against-the-rule cases, a 6-mm incision is used with 0.75 to 1.5 D of astigmatism and a 7-mm incision is used with 1.75 to 2.25 D of astigmatism. Larger amounts of astigmatism are corrected with a corneal relaxing incision opposite the cataract incision.

A more conservative approach is used in with-the-rule cases. Small incisions are used with up to 2 D of with-the-rule astigmatism. For 2 to 2.25 D, a 6-mm incision is used, and for 2.5 to 2.75 D a 7-mm incision is used. For 3 D or more, a corneal relaxing incision is added.

For both with-the-rule and against-the-rule patients, the style of incision also changes based on the astigmatism level and the steepness at the incision site noted on the topography. If a foldable lens is to be inserted, a frown incision is used (Figure 9-1A). With moderate steepness, a tangential incision is used (Figure 9-1B), and with greater steepness a limbus-parallel incision is used (Figure 9-1C).

Surgical Technique

The patient is taken to the holding area where the corneal topography is used to guide marking of the cataract incision. This axis is marked with a surgical marking pen under topical anesthesia. The patient is then given a peribulbar block. The Honan cuff is applied at 30 mmHg for ten minutes. The patient is prepped with 50% Betadine solution. A drape is positioned and a wire lid speculum is inserted.

The cataract incision is placed at the appropriate axis. Construction of the cataract wound is very important. If the topography shows minimal steepness at the cataract wound location, a foldable IOL is used with a frown incision (Figure 9-1A). With progressively greater steepness, the wound is enlarged and placed more parallel to the limbus (Figures 9-1B and 9-1C). However, the wound never exceeds 7 mm in length.

The incision is made entirely with a 3.2-mm keratome (Alcon). The scleral tunnel advances 1.5 mm into the cornea. After squaring off the anterior aspect of the tunnel, I press the keratome down and enter the anterior chamber. If properly constructed, this wound rarely has to be sutured.

Results

A consecutive cohort of 36 cases who received a 6 to 7-mm sutureless cataract incision at or near the steep axis of preoperative cylinder was analyzed. All cases had at least one month postoperative data. Preoperatively, keratometric cylinder ranged from 0.87 D to 4 D with a mean of 1.81 D. Postoperatively, keratometric cylinder ranged from 0 to 2.5 D with a mean of 0.99 D.

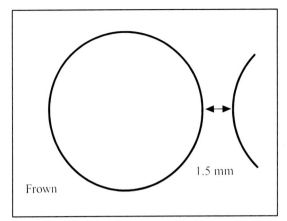

Figure 9-1A. Frown incision for cases with little pre-existing astigmatism.

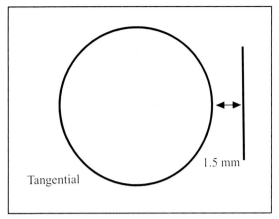

Figure 9-1B. Tangential incision for moderate steepness.

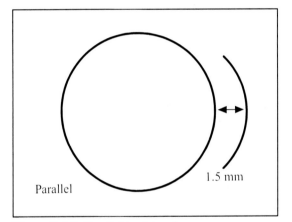

Figure 9-1C. Parallel incision for greater steepness.

Figure 9-1. The center of the cataract incision is always placed 1.5 mm posterior to the limbus. With progressively greater steepness in the incision meridian, the wound is placed more parallel to the limbus.

Figure 9-2 illustrates the amount of cylinder induced 90° away from the preoperative cylinder versus the preoperative cylinder. The induced cylinder was computed using vector analysis methods to account for axis shifts. Points within the dashed lines indicate cases for whom the induced cylinder in the correcting axis was within 0.5 D of preoperative cylinder. Points below the line received only a partial correction of cylinder. Only one case had a significant overcorrection.

Figure 9-3 shows the magnitude of the postoperative versus preoperative cylinder without regard to axis. Two cases had a slight increase in cylinder, fourteen cases were within 0.5 D of their preoperative level, and 20 cases experienced a reduction in astigmatism of more than 0.5 D, some by 2 to 3 D. Cases with more than 2 D of cylinder preoperatively achieved better results than cases with 2 D or less preoperatively. Figure 9-4 shows the distribution of changes in cylinder power for cases with 2 D or less cylinder preoperatively and cases with more than 2 D. Changes were

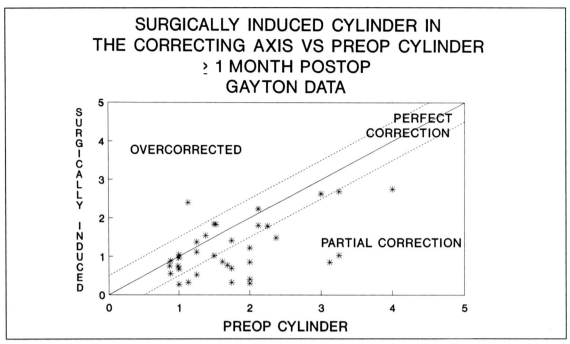

Figure 9-2. Cylinder induced 90° away from the preoperative keratometric cylinder (correcting axis) versus the preoperative cylinder. Points within the dashed lines indicate cases for whom the induced cylinder in the correcting axis was within 0.5 D of preoperative cylinder. Points below the solid line received a partial correction of cylinder, while points above had an overcorrection.

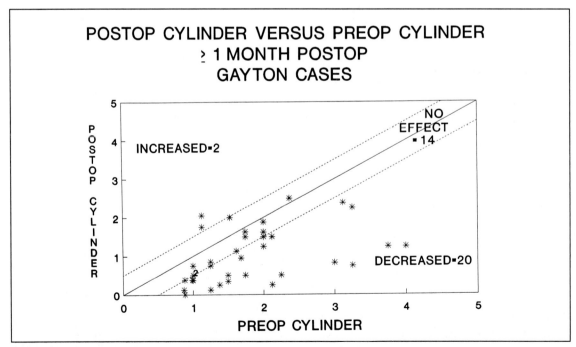

Figure 9-3. Postoperative versus preoperative keratometric cylinder levels. Points within the dashed lines were within 0.5 D of preoperative cylinder postoperatively. Points below the solid line had a decrease in cylinder while points above had an increase.

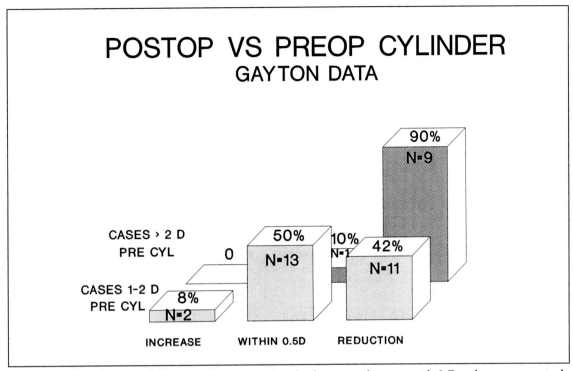

Figure 9-4. Distribution of changes in keratometric cylinder power for cases with 2 D or less preoperatively and cases with more than 2 D.

categorized as an increase in cylinder, a decrease, or essentially no change. All but one case with more than 2 D preoperatively achieved a significant reduction in astigmatism. Among cases with 2 D or less, half had no net change in astigmatism, while two cases had an increase of more than 0.5 D. All but one of the temporal incision cases were either within 0.5 D of preoperative cylinder or substantially reduced (Figure 9-5). Since often against-the-rule cylinder is worsened by traditional superior-incision cataract surgery, this result is quite good. These cases achieved a mean reduction in against-the-rule cylinder of 44%.

Figure 9-6 shows the preoperative versus postoperative axis. Most cases did not experience a major shift in cylinder axis. Some with-the-rule cases shifted to against-the-rule postoperatively. These were early cases before a more conservative approach to with-the-rule cylinder was taken.

Topography of Rotated Cataract Incisions

Figures 9-7A to 9-7C shows the topography of an 84 year-old woman who received a 6-mm scleral-tunnel self-sealing cataract incision which was designed to slip a little postoperatively. Figure 9-7A demonstrates the preoperative and one day postoperative corneal appearance and the surgically induced change. The change image shows some steepening induced where the cornea had been flattest, 90° away from the incision. However, the most prominent change is flattening at the incision site. Figure 9-7B shows the preoperative topography and the surgically caused changes over time. As the temporal wound slipped in the early postoperative period, the cornea gradually steepened superiorly and the temporal flattening resolved. Figure 9-7C shows the one

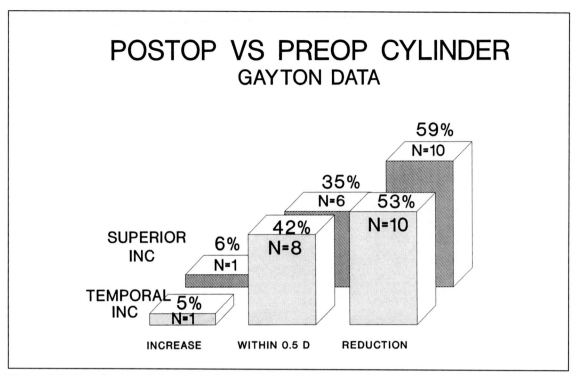

Figure 9-5. Distribution of changes in keratometric cylinder power for cases receiving a temporal cataract incision and cases receiving a superior incision.

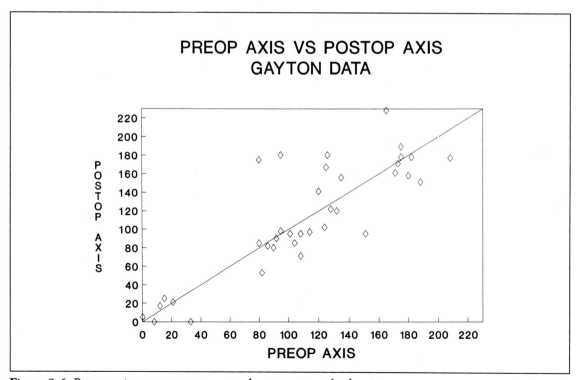

Figure 9-6. Preoperative versus postoperative keratometric cylinder axis.

month topography, demonstrating a relatively spherical central cornea. By this visit, the 1.25 D of preoperative keratometric cylinder had been virtually eliminated.

The Rowan Approach

The Rowan approach is designed to reduce pre-existing astigmatism in the cataract patient while avoiding overcorrections. Rather than use corneal relaxing incisions, which can result in overcorrections and less predictable results, the incision for astigmatic correction is combined with the cataract incision. The technique uses a limbal relaxing incision—a large arcuate incision of three-quarters thickness made about 1 mm posterior to the surgical limbus—centered at the steep axis of astigmatism. The limbal relaxing incision is 60° of arc for small amounts of astigmatism, 90° of arc for moderate amounts of astigmatism, and 120° of arc for three or more diopters of astigmatism. Within the central 3.5 mm of the incision, a tunnel is made for a standard self-sealing entry into the cornea (Figures 9-8A through 9-8C).

Most cataract patients with significant pre-existing astigmatism have the against-the rule type. Thus, the key to the technique, as for any technique that involves making the cataract incision at the steep axis, is the ability to perform the cataract surgery temporally. The change to the temporal approach is actually easily made. In fact, the exposure, the red reflex, and the ease of approach is actually better than with the superior approach.

Surgical Technique

The relaxing incision is made 1 to 1.5 mm posterior to the limbus and parallel with the limbus. The surgeon uses a diamond blade and makes the incision freehand, though any preferred blade could be used, including a guarded or set blade. The initial incision should be approximately 3/4 scleral depth. This incision is then undermined or "stepped" into a two-plane incision, very much the same as though a planned extracapsular incision was being made (Figure 9-8A). The incision does not enter the anterior chamber at this point.

The first part of the incision is made nearly perpendicular to the scleral surface, and to approximately 3/4 scleral depth. The second step of the incision is oriented approximately 90° to the first, following the plane of the sclera. This second part is started with the same small diamond blade. It is then further undermined with a pocket or tunnel-type round, flat blade. Attention is given to freely undermining the incision at this point so that the incised sclera will be able to relax and "kick up" noticeably. Dissection is carried part way up into clear cornea in the center of the incision, though still without entering the anterior chamber. This undermining portion of the incision design needs to be thorough if significant astigmatism reduction is to be accomplished. The relaxation observed at this point is essentially what will be obtained ("what you see is what you get"), so attention needs to be given to this undermining step. A limbal incision of 60° is used for a target of 1 D, 90° for a target of 2 D, and 120° for 3 D or more. The final step in making the incision is the clear-corneal, self-sealing anterior chamber entry, which is made in the middle of the incision (Figures 9-8B and 9-8C). A keratome or a 15° blade can be used to make this 3.5-mm incision.

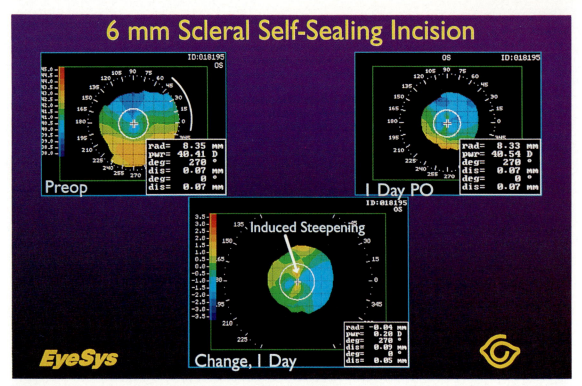

Figure 9-7A. Preoperative (upper left), one day postoperative (upper right), and change map images demonstrating slight steepening superiorly and flattening at the incision site.

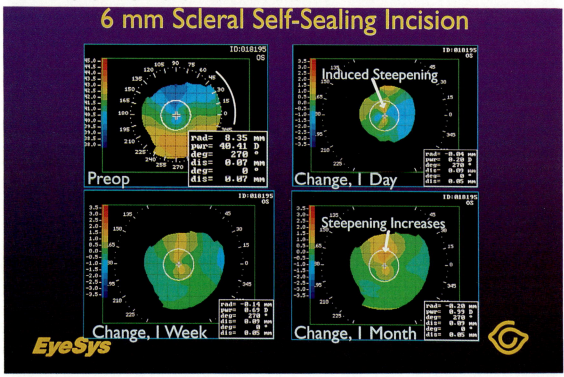

Figure 9-7B. Preoperative and one day, one week, and one month change map images demonstrating gradual increase of superior steepening and resolution of the flattening at the incision site.

Figure 9-7. Corneal topography of a patient who received a temporal 6-mm scleral-tunnel sutureless cataract incision which was designed to slip.

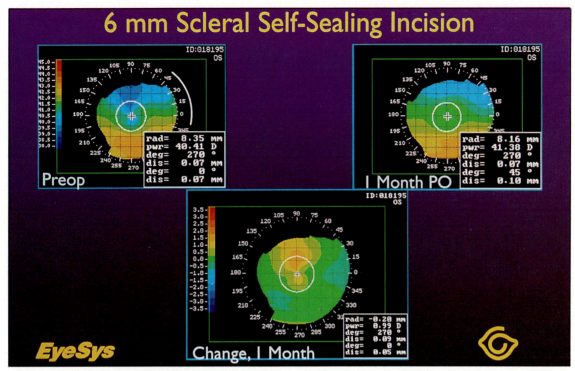

Figure 9-7C. Preoperative, one month postoperative, and change map images.

Results

A consecutive cohort of 54 cases receiving a limbal relaxing incision combined with a 3.5-mm cataract incision was analyzed. All cases had three month postoperative data. Preoperative keratometric cylinder ranged from 0.63 to 3.5 D, with a mean of 1.51 D. Astigmatic correction between 1 and 3 D was targeted, although most cases (81%) were targeted for 1 to 1.5 D of correction.

Postoperatively, keratometric cylinder ranged from 0.25 to 3.0 D, with a mean of 1.10 D. The mean percent correction of cylinder was 48.8%. Figure 9-9 demonstrates the amount of cylinder that was induced in a direction to counteract preoperative cylinder (the correcting axis) versus the preoperative level of astigmatism. Points falling within the dashed lines demonstrate cases that had within 0.5 D of a perfect correction, that is, induced cylinder in the correcting axis equal to preoperative cylinder. While many cases had essentially a perfect correction, most cases were undercorrected. Only one case was significantly overcorrected.

Figure 9-10 shows the postoperative versus preoperative level of cylinder without regard to axis. Although many cases had essentially no change in cylinder level, most cases had a reduction of greater than 0.25 D.

For the most part, these cases did not experience axis shifts in their cylinder. Figure 9-11 displays the preoperative versus postoperative cylinder axis. Most cases were against-the-rule preoperatively and remained so postoperatively. Three cases shifted from against-the-rule to with-the-rule.

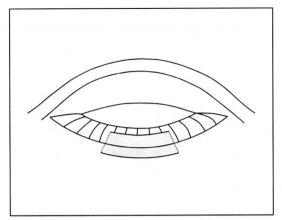

Figure 9-8A. Arcuate incision at the steep axis approximately 1 mm posterior to the limbus, which is undermined into a two-plane incision about 3/4 depth.

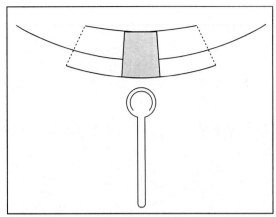

Figure 9-8B. Within the central 3.5 mm of the incision, a tunnel is extended into clear cornea with a pocket blade.

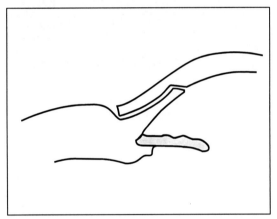

Figure 9-8C. A corneal lip is created to make a self-sealing entry.

Figure 9-8. Construction of limbal relaxing cataract incision.

Topography of Limbal Relaxing Cataract Incisions

Figure 9-12 shows topography of a case who received a limbal relaxing incision and self-sealing cataract incision. Preoperatively, the case had 2.5 D of with-the-rule astigmatism, so the incision was centered at 80°. The surgery did result in a correction of some of the astigmatism as seen in the one day postoperative image. The change image on the bottom shows the induced change. There was flattening in the meridian of the incision, with steepening 90° away.

Figure 9-13 shows topography of a case with 1.5 D of against-the-rule astigmatism preoperatively who received a temporal limbal relaxing cataract incision centered at 15°. The change image shows flattening in the incision meridian and steepening 90° away, resulting in good correction of the astigmatism.

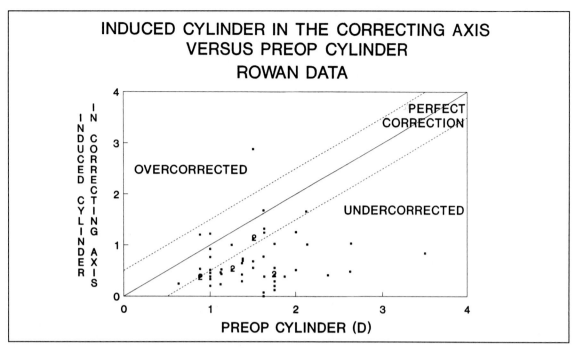

Figure 9-9. Cylinder induced 90° away from the preoperative keratometric cylinder (correcting axis) versus the preoperative cylinder. Points within the dashed lines indicate cases for whom the induced cylinder in the correcting axis was within 0.5 D of preoperative cylinder. Points below the solid line received a partial correction of cylinder, while points above had an overcorrection.

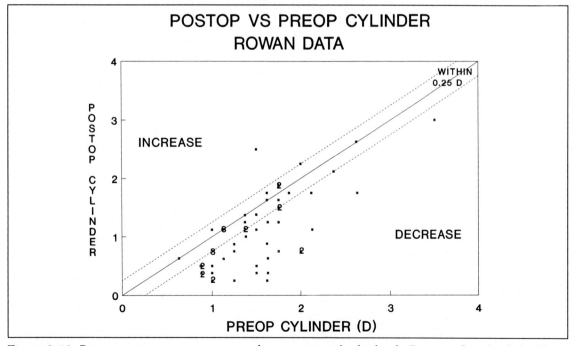

Figure 9-10. Postoperative versus preoperative keratometric cylinder levels. Points within the dashed lines were within 0.25 D of preoperative cylinder postoperatively. Points below the solid line had a decrease in cylinder while points above had an increase.

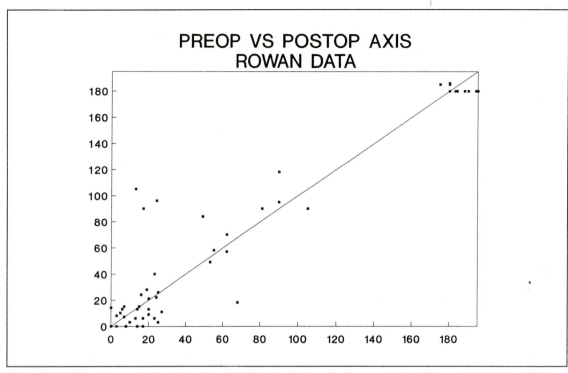

Figure 9-11. Preoperative versus postoperative keratometric cylinder axis. Vertical axis is postoperative axis and horizontal axis is preoperative axis.

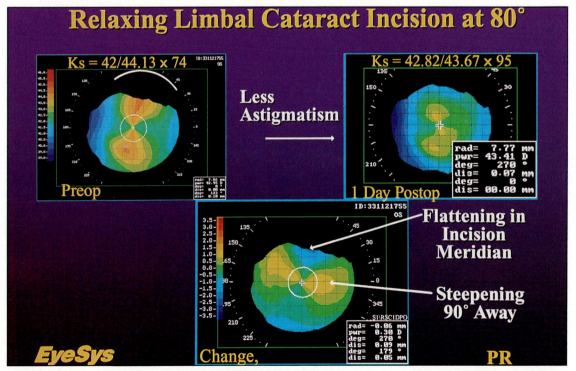

Figure 9-12. One day postoperative result following a relaxing limbal cataract incision at 80°.

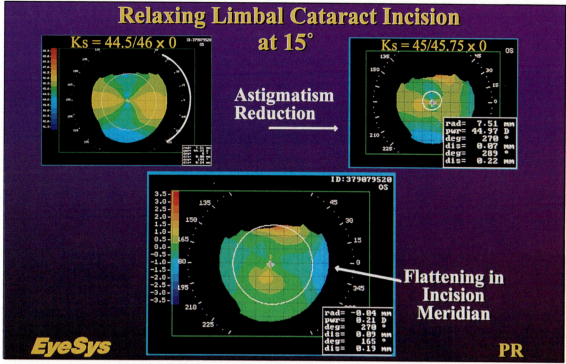

Figure 9-13. Result of a relaxing limbal cataract incision at 15°.

Figure 9-14 shows a case with 4.5 D of against-the-rule cylinder preoperatively. Such a case is not correctable from the superior limbus, and would require very aggressive astigmatic keratotomy incisions. The patient received a temporal limbal relaxing cataract incision of 120° of arc. The incision produced a lot of flattening in the incision meridian, especially at the wound site. The astigmatism was essentially neutralized overnight.

Discussion

There are a number of different techniques for correcting pre-existing cylinder in cataract cases: wound management techniques; corneal relaxing incisions, which are discussed in Chapter 3; and the toric intraocular lens, which is discussed in Chapter 11. No one technique is necessarily the best for every patient. Surgeon and/or patient preferences, patient characteristics, and preoperative level of cylinder may all be factors affecting the most appropriate choice of surgical technique for a patient.

The two techniques covered in this chapter use entirely different strategies to manage astigmatism, with different results. The Gayton approach, which is to use a larger cataract incision, may be more appropriate for patients with moderate levels of astigmatism. The Rowan approach, which uses an undermined limbal relaxing incision combined with a small cataract incision, may be best for patients with low levels of cylinder. Other wound management techniques have been

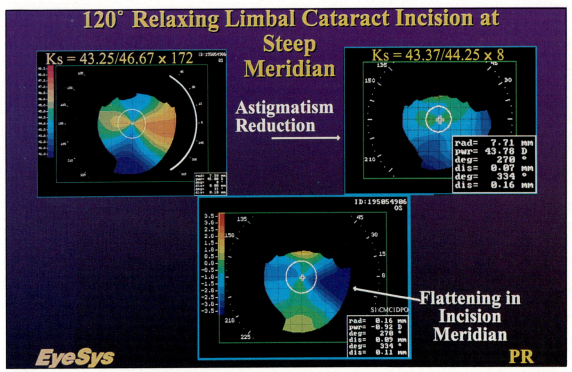

Figure 9-14. One day postoperative result following a temporal, relaxing limbal cataract incision of 120° of arc for correction of 4.5 D of against-the-rule astigmatism.

described in the past, or may be under investigation now, each with their own inherent advantages and disadvantages.

What these techniques share is the use of the cataract incision to minimize the astigmatism postoperatively. This strategy involves placing the incision at the steep axis, which requires the surgeon to be flexible in his surgical technique and adjust to new positions. Inevitably, the surgeon will experience a learning curve, but many surgeons who have tried these techniques consider the results worth the additional effort.

References

1. Gills JP: Football mnemonic for correction of preoperative astigmatism. *Am Intra-Ocular Implant Soc J* 9:57, 1983

2. Maloney W, Grindle L: Surgically tailored astigmatism reduction (STAR). In *Textbook of Phacoemulsification.* Fallbrook, CA, Lasenda Publishers, pp 85-106, 1988.

3. Maloney WF: STAR approach: surgically tailored astigmatism reduction. In Gills JP, Sanders DR, eds, *Small-Incision Cataract Surgery: Foldable Lenses, One-Stitch Surgery, Sutureless Surgery, Astigmatic Keratotomy.* Thorofare, NJ, SLACK, Inc., pp 177-189, 1990.

10

Keratolenticuloplasty

ROBERT M. KERSHNER, MD

Introduction

Cataract surgery has undergone a phenomenal change over the past decade. At one time in-patient hospitalization, general anesthesia, large surgical incisions, multiple sutures, and aphakic spectacle correction postoperatively was considered the norm. Gradually cataract surgeons improved cataract removal techniques allowing better visual rehabilitation with intraocular lens implantation. Careful selection of small incision one-piece and three-piece IOLs made IOL implantation possible without significantly altering astigmatism. In time, surgical techniques evolved from large incision extracapsular extraction with sutures to sutureless small incision phacoemulsification, minimizing iatrogenically-induced astigmatism from the procedure. However, pre-existing refractive errors, including astigmatism and presbyopia, continue to persist as the number one indication for postoperative spectacle correction.

Spherical errors are correctable with careful and accurate preoperative ultrasonic biometry and appropriate intraocular lens implant with bifocal capability. However pre-existing astigmatic errors continue to plague the cataract surgeon. Recent advances in the corneal approach to cataract surgery have created the opportunity for the surgeon to take advantage of the corneal incision placement to fully correct the refractive error of the patient at the time of cataract extraction, providing the best uncorrected visual acuity postoperatively. I named this procedure keratolenticuloplasty (KLP) to reflect the remodeling of the cornea and the replacement of the lens through a corneal incision to achieve emmetropia.

There are compelling reasons to correct refractive errors. First is patient preference and lifestyle. Freedom to be able to drive, work, read, swim, and play without dependence on spectacle or contact lenses is a normal desire. Second is economic. In the United States alone over three billion dollars a year is spent on eyewear (glasses and contact lenses).

Eliminating dependence on these appliances will save the consumer hundreds of millions of dollars in doctor's visits, refractions, fitting and dispensing of eyewear. The number one refractive procedure performed in the United States today is cataract surgery. Therefore, all cataract surgeons are *de facto* refractive surgeons. The recent advances in the technology of computer-assisted videokeratography (corneal topography), finely calibrated keratomes for corneal incisions, and precision methods of measuring corneal thickness (ultrasonic pachymetry) have provided the refractive surgeon with superior tools for achieving precise and reproducible refractive corrections. Today we have the ability to correct all forms of refractive error with combined cataract and refractive surgery.

Keratolenticuloplasty—The Procedure

Surgeons should be wary of those who claim that they perform one cataract incision technique "100% of the time." There is no single approach to cataract surgery which is ideal for all patients. Today's technological advances and instrumentation allow us to use a "tailor-made" approach to surgery. Surgeons who are undertaking refractive cataract surgery should be well versed in small-incision cataract surgery, capsulorhexis, hydrodissection, and in-the-bag phaco-emulsification and small incision intraocular lens implantation.[1-3] Knowledge and use of topical anesthesia is helpful, although not mandatory. Topical anesthesia techniques have been well covered elsewhere.[4-6]

The key to this procedure is careful preoperative keratometry of the cornea and meticulous ultrasonic biometry to determine the proper spherical correction to be provided by the intraocular lens implant. A complete examination of the eye with attention to the cornea to screen for scars or irregularity is important. Cycloplegic refraction and evaluation of the preoperative computerized topography enables the surgeon to identify the axis of steepest astigmatism (which sometimes may be quite asymmetrical). A surgical plan can then be constructed.

Incision construction is the key to a self-sealing and rapidly healing incision. The anatomy and architecture of scleral-tunnel and clear-corneal incisions have been discussed extensively elsewhere.[3,6] Scleral-tunnel incisions can be almost completely astigmatically neutral in that they do not induce iatrogenic astigmatism. They are, however, incapable of correcting pre-existing astigmatism. Clear-corneal incisions properly constructed can be minimally astigmatic. Arcuate corneal incisions which parallel the optical zone induce the most flattening, and reverse curve (frown) induce the least. The incision's tendency to alter corneal curvature can be utilized to correct pre-existing astigmatic errors.

Clear-corneal incisions can be combined with an arcuate keratotomy to maximize the astigmatic correcting potential of the incision. Arcuate corneal incisions have been well described by Dr. Spencer Thornton and others.[7-9] Arcuate corneal incisions exert greater effect for less surgery because they exactly follow the radius of the optical zone. Arcuate incisions have the same chord length as a simple straight transverse incision. However, they exert about 20% greater effect in changing corneal curvature than straight incisions. I therefore use arcuate incisions for the correction of astigmatism and make all transverse corneal incisions (cataract, astigmatic, etc.) as arcuate incisions.

I classify cataract incisions into three categories:

1. *Scleral-tunnel incisions* when no pre-existing astigmatism is present (40% of cataract procedures).

2. *Single clear-corneal incisions* placed on the steepest axis of astigmatism to correct small amounts of astigmatism (30% of cataract procedures).

3. *Paired arcuate keratotomy incisions* for correcting large degrees of pre-existing astigmatism (approximately 30% of cataract procedures).

If the preoperative astigmatic cylinder is 1 D or less, then a 2.5-mm to 3-mm scleral-tunnel incision can be utilized. If the preoperative astigmatic cylinder is one diopter or greater, then an arcuate clear-corneal keratotomy is utilized for the cataract incision. Astigmatic powers greater than 1.50 D can be corrected with a combined approach of clear-corneal arcuate keratotomy and a paired arcuate keratotomy opposite the cataract incision. The incisions are placed to correspond to the steepest axis of astigmatism as determined by preoperative topography. In many instances the axis of astigmatism is not symmetrical, and therefore the arcuate incisions are positioned to correspond to the steepest axis of each arm of astigmatism. Arcuate incisions are placed 2.5 mm to 4.5 mm from the optical center of the cornea according to the nomogram for the correction desired (in diopters). In most cases of keratolenticuloplasty, either a single 2.5-mm arcuate keratotomy at the 8 to 9-mm optical zone or a pair of 2.5-mm incisions at the 7 to 8-mm optical zone will be all that is required.

The computerized topographic maps are used in the operating room and positioned next to the patient. An astigmatic axis reticule is installed in the operating microscope ocular and the microscope positioned perpendicular over the patient's eye to be able to center the optical zone and identify the axis of the cylinder during the procedure.

Intraoperative keratometry may be helpful but is not necessary if the microscope is properly positioned and the topography consulted during the procedure. Ultrasonic pachymetry is performed at the site of the planned incision. The patient is asked to look into the microscope light. The optical zone is marked with the appropriate marker (Figures 10-1 and 10-2) and, simultaneously, the arcuate incision(s) positioned corresponding to the steepest meridian of the astigmatism (Figure 10-3). The diamond keratome is set to 100% of pachymetry (Figure 10-4) and calibrated under a microscope. The arcuate incisions are then created with the keratome (Figure 10-5A and 10-5B). The length of the incision will correspond to the magnitude of the correction required.

A gentle clockwise rotation of the keratome handle between the thumb and the index finger allows the blade to track in an arcuate manner. Two arcuate incisions are then created.

The arcuate incision closest to the surgeon is utilized for the entry into the anterior chamber. Using a 2.5-mm diamond trifaceted keratome positioned perpendicular to the base of the arcuate keratotomy, a 1.25-mm horizontal corneal track is created at the depth of the arcuate incision (Figure 10-6), leaving approximately 85 microns of tissue at the base of the incision and a 1.25-mm "tunnel" into the anterior chamber. The 2.5-mm keratotomy allows phacoemulsification and injection of a single piece silicone IOL into the capsular bag (Figure 10-7). No sutures or bandage contact lenses are used and the eye is not bandaged at the conclusion of the procedure (Figure 10-8). Postoperative antibiotic and anti-inflammatory drops (such as TobraDex, Tobramycin, Dexamethasone solution) are started and continued four times a day for ten days.

Figures 10-9 through 10-12 demonstrate the topographic changes induced by clear-corneal incisions and arcuate keratotomy incisions.

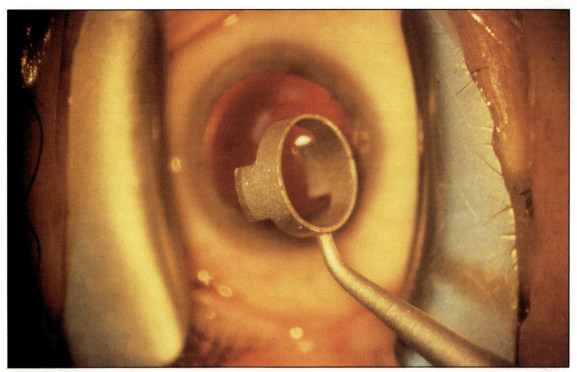

Figure 10-1. Side profile of Kershner arcuate marker.

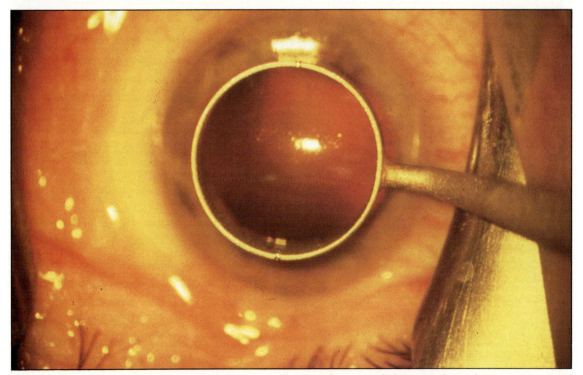

Figure 10-2. The marker is positioned to center the optical zone and the arcs along the steepest axis of astigmatism.

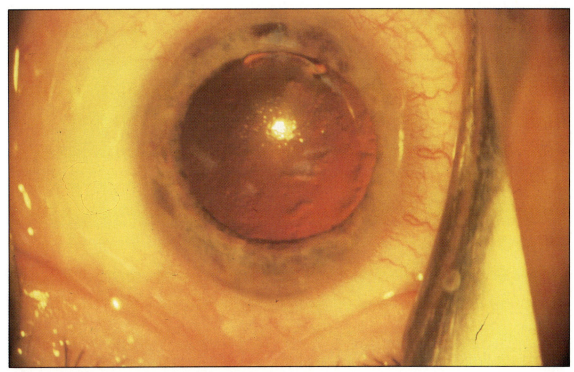

Figure 10-3. Two 3-mm arcuate marks are created.

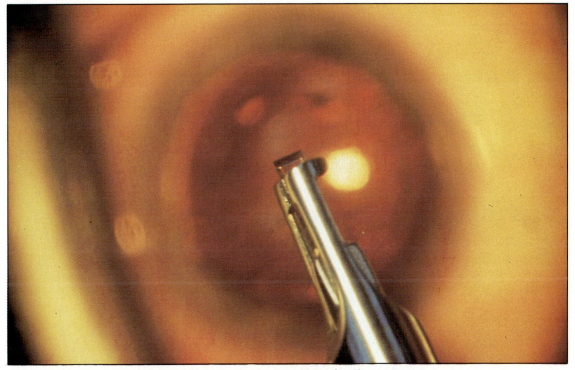

Figure 10-4. The arcuate diamond keratome is set to 100% of pachymetry.

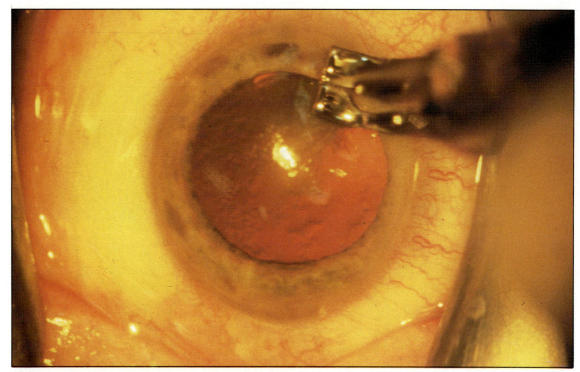

Figure 10-5A. The initial arcuate incision is incised.

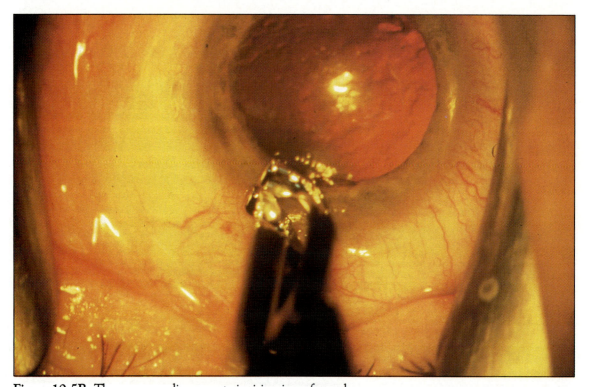

Figure 10-5B. The corresponding arcuate incision is performed.

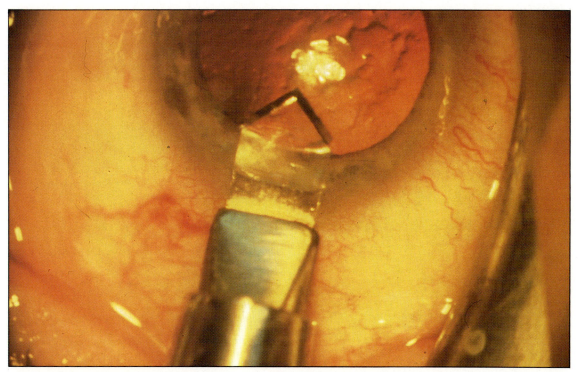

Figure 10-6. A 2.5-mm diamond keratome is placed perpendicular to the base of the arcuate incision closest to the surgeon, entering the anterior chamber 1.25 mm distal to the keratotomy. This creates a two step clear-corneal incision which is self sealing.

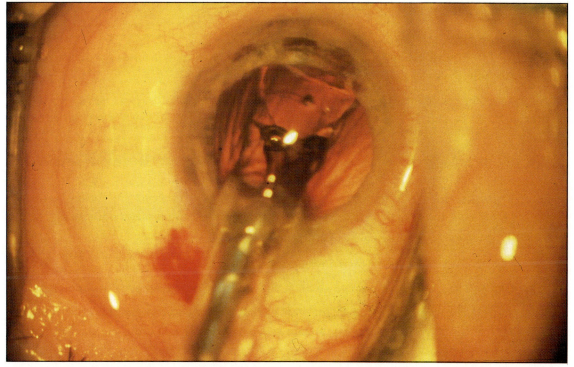

Figure 10-7. A 2.5-mm injection cartridge is used to insert a one-piece elastic lens into the capsular bag.

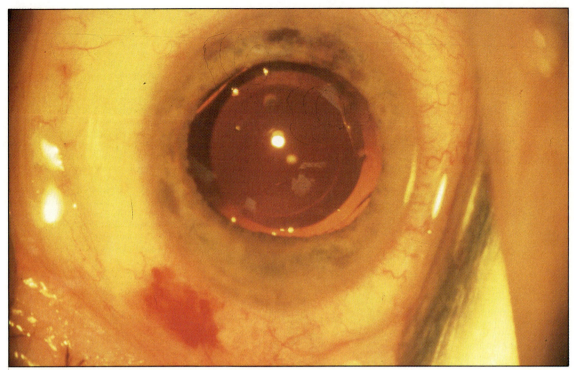

Figure 10-8. The intraocular lens at the conclusion of surgery. The arcuate keratotomy incision does not interfere with visualization.

Nomogram

When the surgeon elects to perform keratolenticuloplasty, certain rules should be kept in mind. I call these the caveats of KLP.

1. Always slightly undercorrect the pre-existing astigmatism. You can always do more surgery later if needed, but it may be difficult to undo what you have already done if you have done too much.

2. It is best to avoid arcuate incisions inside the 7-mm optical zone. That is, if possible, it is preferable to achieve the same degree of correction at 7 mm with a slightly larger arc than to make a smaller arc at a 6-mm optical zone. In other words, incisions are always better the further away from the optical zone they are placed even though their effect decreases.

3. Arcuate incisions should never exceed 90° in length at any optical zone.

4. 85% of depth is ideal for an astigmatic effect.

5. Whenever possible, if a single arcuate incision will suffice it is preferable to two incisions.

6. Always attempt to keep the arcuate incision closest to the surgeon for the entry into the anterior chamber at the limbal vascular arcade at 9, 8 or 7 mm. Avoid using the arcuate incision for the subsequent cataract surgery if it is closer to the optical center of the eye than the 7-mm optical zone.

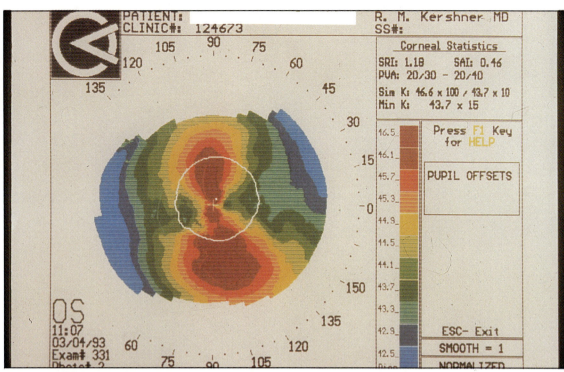

Figure 10-9A. Preoperative topography of with-the-rule astigmatism.

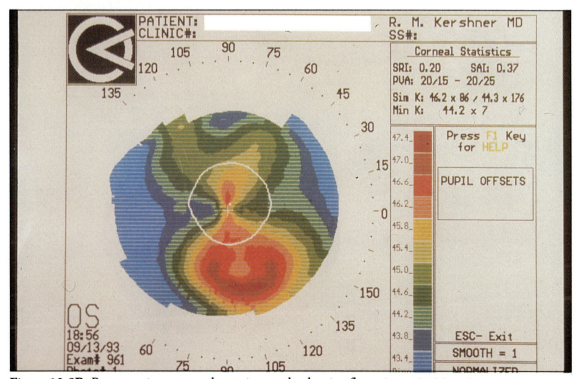

Figure 10-9B. Postoperative topography at six months showing flattening at incision site.

Figure 10-9. Case of with-the-rule astigmatism preoperatively receiving a clear-corneal arcuate incision at 95°.

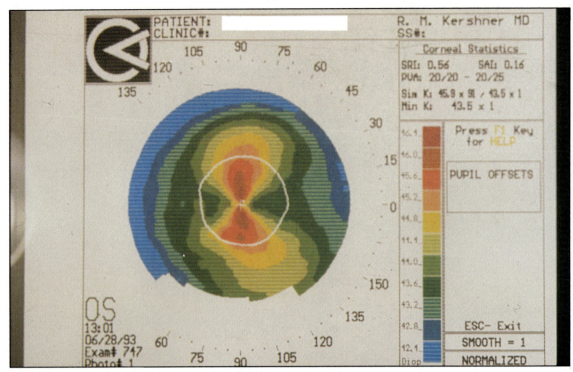

Figure 10-10A. Preoperative topography of with-the-rule astigmatism.

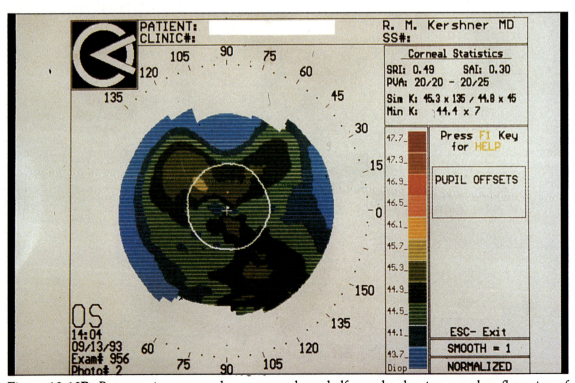

Figure 10-10B. Postoperative topography at two and one-half months showing complete flattening of astigmatism.

Figure 10-10. Case of with-the-rule astigmatism receiving a pair of arcuate keratotomy incisions.

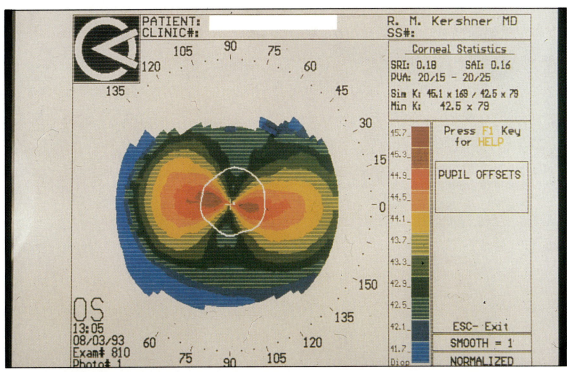

Figure 10-11A. Preoperative topography of against-the-rule astigmatism.

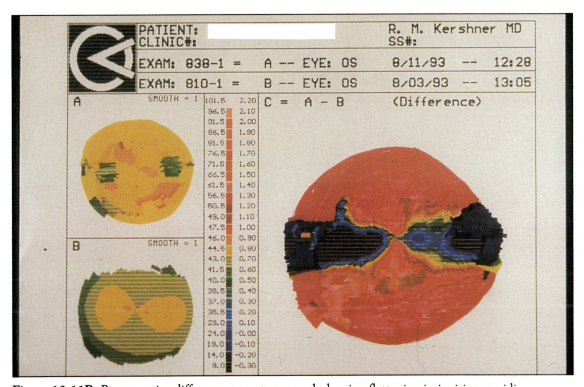

Figure 10-11B. Postoperative difference map at one week showing flattening in incision meridian.

Figure 10-11. Case with against-the-rule astigmatism receiving a pair of arcuate keratotomy incisions.

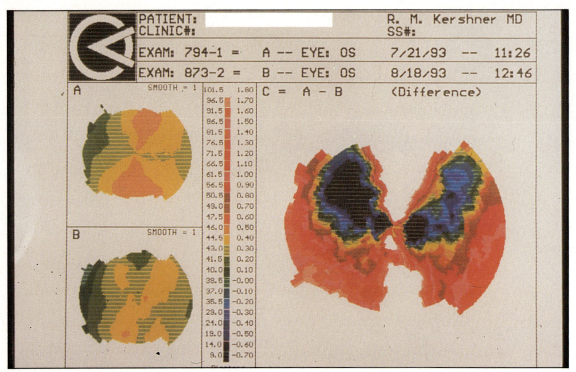

Figure 10-12. Difference map at three weeks postoperatively with paired arcuate incisions at 90°.

7. To avoid full thickness penetration, avoid pressing on the globe with another instrument during the creation of the arcuate incision. Holding the eye, if required at all, is best performed with a toothed forceps.

8. It is easier to visualize the marks and incise the cornea if the cornea is kept slightly dry.

9. Avoid using marking inks. They obscure visualization for subsequent procedures during the surgery. A clean marker gently pressed onto the epithelium will create a visible mark that will be more than satisfactory as a guideline to creating the incision.

10. Simply placing the corneal cataract incision on the axis of steepest astigmatism will almost always improve the refractive result. However, operating on the incorrect axis will usually make the refractive result worse. Axis is crucial.

The nomogram (Table 10-1) is designed to be used with the Kershner One-Step Arcuate Keratotomy system which includes a triple-edge diamond keratome and set of 3-mm arcuate keratotomy markers with optical zones of 5, 6, 7, 8, and 9 mm. The nomogram is to be used strictly as a guideline. Each individual surgeon should modify his or her values based upon the results obtained in her or his hands.

Table 10-1.
Kershner Arcuate Keratotomy System Nomogram

Correction (Diopters)	Optical Zone (mm)	Arcuate Incision Length (mm)
1.0	9 mm	2.5 mm (1)
1.5	8 mm	2.0 mm
2.0	8 mm	2.5 mm
2.5	7 mm	2.5 mm
3.0	7 mm	3.0 mm
3.5	7 mm	3.0 mm
4.0	6 mm	2.0 mm
4.5	6 mm	2.5 mm
5.0	6 mm	3.0 mm
5.5	5 mm	2.0 mm
6.0	5 mm	2.5 mm

Corrected for age 60+. Arcs placed on steepest axis of astigmatism (plus cylinder). Pachymetry at incision site, square diamond keratome set to 100% of pachymetry. Mark arcuate incisions and optical zone with Kershner One-Step Marker.

Summary

Arcuate keratotomy combined with cataract surgery is one of the most powerful techniques for the permanent correction for pre-existing refractive errors that we have today. Take the time to study it carefully and master it well. With experience, it will become one of the most satisfying aspects of your surgical practice.

References

1. Kershner RM: A new one step forceps for capsulorhexis. *J Cataract Refract Surg* 16:762-767, 1990.

2. Kershner RM: Embryology, anatomy and needle capsulotomy. In Koch PS, Davison JA, eds, *Textbook of Phacoemulsification Techniques*, Thorofare, NJ, SLACK, Inc., pp. 35-48, 1990.

3. Kershner RM: Sutureless one handed intercapsular phacoemulsification - the keyhole technique. *J Cataract Refract Surg* 17 (supplement):719-725, 1991.

4. Kershner RM: No stitch topical anesthesia. In Gills JP, Hustead RF, Sanders DR, eds, *Ophthalmic Anesthesia*, Thorofare, NJ, SLACK, Inc., pp. 172-175, 1993.

5. Kershner RM: Topical anesthesia for small incision self sealing cataract surgery-a prospective study of the first 100 patients. *J Cataract Refract Surg* 19:290-292, 1993.

6. Kershner RM: Topical anesthesia cataract surgery. In Fine IH, Fichman RA, Grabow HB, eds, *Clear-Corneal Cataract Surgery*, Thorofare, NJ, SLACK, Inc., pp. 141-153, 1993.

7. Rowsey JJ: Review: current concepts in astigmatism surgery. *J Refract Surg* 2:85-94, 1986.

8. Thornton SP: Astigmatic keratotomy with cataract extraction: Thornton nomogram for quantitative surgery. In Gills JP, Sanders DR, eds, *Small-Incision Cataract Surgery: Foldable Lenses, One-Stitch Surgery, Sutureless Surgery, Astigmatic Keratotomy*, Thorofare, NJ, SLACK, Inc., pp. 245-258, 1990.

9. Thornton SP: Theory behind corneal relaxing incisions/Thornton nomogram. In Gills JP, Martin RG, Sanders DR, eds, *Sutureless Cataract Surgery: An Evolution Toward Minimally Invasive Technique*, Thorofare, NJ, SLACK, Inc., pp. 123-143, 1992.

Section IV

Intraocular Lens Correction

11

Clinical Investigation of a Toric IOL: FDA Study Update

Donald R. Sanders, MD, PhD
Manus C. Kraff, MD
John Shepherd, MD
Harry B. Grabow, MD

Introduction

Until now, surgical correction of pre-existing astigmatism in cataract surgery has involved corneal relaxing incisions, rotated cataract incisions, posterior versus anterior placement of the wound, suture type and placement, modification of incision length, or some combination. The potential clinical problems associated with these techniques include weakened corneal structure, corneal perforations, lack of predictability of effect, and regression of effect. With the advent of astigmatically neutral cataract surgery associated with small incision IOLs, the incorporation of a toric correction onto a silicone lens implant is a natural progression towards the elimination of pre-existing astigmatism. The first clinical investigation of such a device is being conducted by STAAR Surgical Company (Monrovia, CA) in the United States under the auspices of the FDA.

Study Design and Surgical Technique

Inclusion criteria restrict entry into the study to cataract patients without any previous ocular surgery and who have 2 to 4 D of pre-existing astigmatism as determined in the IOL plane. Determination of astigmatism in the plane of the IOL is accomplished using a modern IOL power formula to compute the two IOL powers corresponding to the curvatures of the steepest and flattest corneal meridians, as opposed to the traditional approach which uses the average corneal curvature to determine the appropriate IOL power choice. The difference between the two IOL powers so determined yields the magnitude of the pre-existing astigmatism in the plane of the IOL. The lens implant used in this study is of one-piece construction and composed entirely of silicone as shown in Figure 11-1.

A randomized, prospective design has been chosen for this investigation to allow for comparison to a suitable control group. Patients fulfilling the inclusion criteria are assigned to either the study group or the control group according to the randomization schedule. Those patients assigned to the study group receive an IOL having +2 D of toric correction incorporated onto the anterior surface of the lens with cylinder axis oriented along the longitudinal axis of the IOL (model AA-4203T). Patients assigned to the control group receive a similar lens design having no toric correction (AA-4203V).

It is important to emphasize that, for the purposes of this study, only a single toric correction is being used. At this point in time, the objective is to demonstrate that the toric IOL produces a systematic reduction in refractive cylinder. As a result, it is anticipated from the outset that patients having greater than 2 D of astigmatism in the IOL plane will be undercorrected.

The cataract surgical technique used in this study includes either scleral-tunnel or clear-corneal incisions of a sutureless construction, followed by capsulorhexis, phacoemulsification and insertion of the IOL into the capsular bag with the Softrans® injector (STAAR Surgical

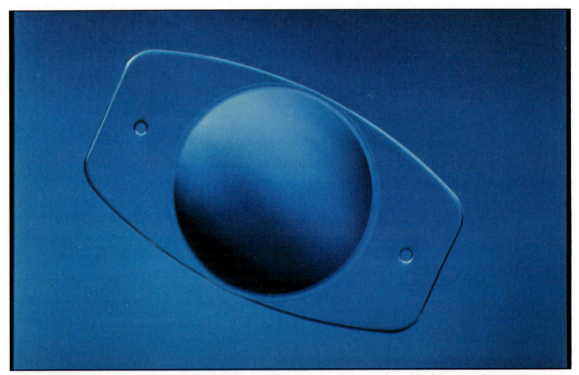

Figure 11-1. STAAR model AA-4203 IOL, which serves as the template for delivery of toric correction into the posterior chamber following cataract surgery.

Company). In the study group, a marking device is applied to the cornea and the lens is rotated such that the longitudinal axis of the IOL is aligned with the axis of steepest corneal curvature as determined preoperatively from keratometry or corneal topography.

Phase I of the investigation is currently underway and will enroll 125 patients in each of the study and control groups. An additional 625 patients will be enrolled into the study group in Phase II pending consent of the FDA.

Clinical Results

Postoperative rotational stability of the toric IOL is important for optimal efficiency in reducing pre-existing astigmatism. Theoretically, a rotation of greater than 30° from the desired axis would increase the patient's refractive cylinder.[1] However, as shown in Figure 11-2, measurements of the postoperative IOL axis demonstrate that 94% of toric patients have experienced IOL rotations of less than 30°.

Both groups have 94% of cases with 20/40 or better corrected acuity. Preoperatively 6% of control patients presented with corneal endothelial disease (guttata), 15% with macular degeneration, and 3% with glaucoma. Preoperatively 2% of study patients presented with endothelial disease (guttata), 18% with macular degeneration, and 4% with glaucoma. All best case patients achieved a corrected acuity of 20/40 or better.

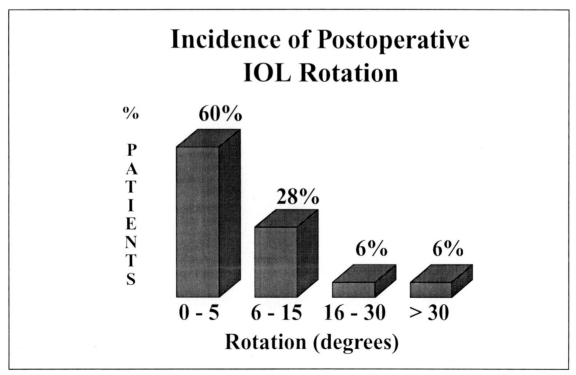

Figure 11-2. Distribution of postoperative rotation of the toric IOL among study patients. Ninety-four percent of patients experienced rotations of less than 30°.

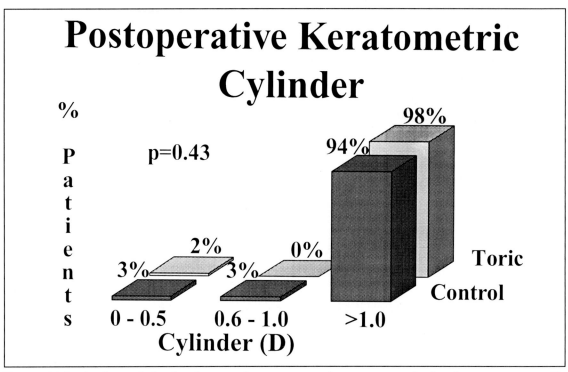

Figure 11-3. Analysis of the distribution of postoperative keratometric cylinder shows no statistically significant difference between study and control patients.

As expected in a randomized investigation involving identical surgical techniques, the distribution of postoperative keratometric cylinder is similar in the study and control groups (Figure 11-3). Despite the equivalence of keratometric cylinder between the groups, Figure 11-4 clearly demonstrates a statistically significant reduction in postoperative refractive cylinder among study patients as a result of implantation of the toric IOL. Thirty-six percent (36%) of toric versus only 9% of control patients have less than or equal to 0.5 D of refractive cylinder. The 42% of study patients having greater than 1.0 D of refractive cylinder shown in Figure 11-4 are a direct manifestation of the fact that the toric IOL is currently available with only one toric correction, as discussed earlier. In the future, if the toric power can be selected based on the pre-existing astigmatism, the incidence of postoperative refractive cylinder of greater than 1.0 D is expected to be even further reduced.

As shown in Figure 11-5 the study group has better uncorrected acuity at each of three levels used for comparison. Further, the increased incidence of 20/40 or better in the study group is already statistically significant (69% versus 40%, p=0.02). The differences in the incidence of 20/30 or better and 20/25 or better between the groups seems to be approaching statistical significance (53% versus 28%, p=0.05 and 25% versus 8%, p=0.09, respectively). The differences in uncorrected vision are not due to differences in spherical refraction, since the postoperative spherical equivalent in both groups is virtually identical (0.45 D versus 0.46 D)

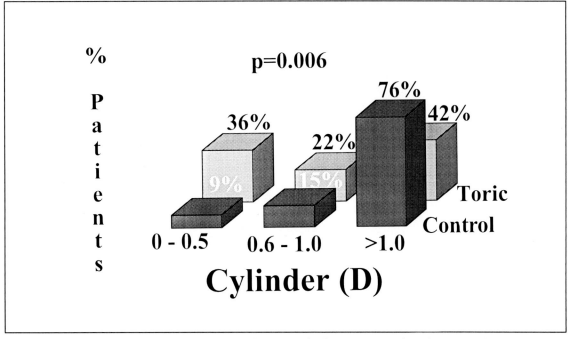

Figure 11-4. Distributions of postoperative refractive cylinder as measured in the spectacle plane for the study and control groups. Analysis demonstrates a statistically significant reduction in cylinder among patients implanted with the toric IOL.

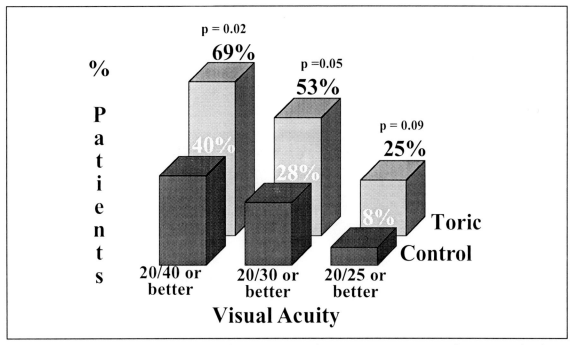

Figure 11-5. Comparison of uncorrected acuity among best case patients using three acuity levels. A statistically significant enhancement in the incidence of 20/40 or better can be observed among toric patients. Further, one in four (25%) of the toric patients achieved 20/25 versus only 8% in the control group.

Conclusion

Based on early clinical results, the STAAR toric IOL for the correction of pre-existing astigmatism shows great promise. The lens already demonstrates a statistically significant decrease in refractive cylinder and improvement in uncorrected acuity when compared to the identical IOL without a toric optic. Final evaluation of the safety and efficacy of this device, however, awaits conclusion of this investigation.

Reference

1. Sanders DR, Grabow HB, Shepherd J, Raanan MG: STAAR AA 4203T toric silicone IOL. In Martin RG, Gills JP, Sanders DR, eds., *Foldable Intraocular Lenses*. Thorofare, NJ, SLACK, Inc., pp 237-250, 1993.

Index